The Role of **Purchasers and Payers** in the **Clinical Research Enterprise**

WORKSHOP SUMMARY

Sean Tunis, Allan Korn, and Alex Ommaya, Editors

Based on a Workshop of the Clinical Research Roundtable

Board on Health Sciences Policy

INSTITUTE OF MEDICINE

NATIONAL ACADEMY PRESS
Washington, D.C.

NATIONAL ACADEMY PRESS • 2101 Constitution Avenue, N.W. • Washington, DC 20418

NOTICE: The project that is the subject of this report was approved by the Governing Board of the National Research Council, whose members are drawn from the councils of the National Academy of Sciences, the National Academy of Engineering, and the Institute of Medicine. The members of the committee responsible for the report were chosen for their special competences and with regard for appropriate balance.

Support for this project was provided by Agency for Healthcare Research and Quality, American Medical Association, Association of American Medical Colleges, BlueCross/BlueShield Association, Burroughs Wellcome Fund, Centers for Disease Control and Prevention, Centers for Medicare and Medicaid Services (formerly HCFA), Department of Veterans Affairs, Doris Duke Charitable Foundation, Food and Drug Administration, Johnson & Johnson, Merck and Company, National Institutes of Health, Pfizer, Inc., and the Robert Wood Johnson Foundation. The views presented in this report are those of the authors and are not necessarily those of the funding agencies.

International Standard Book Number 0-309-08349-0

Library of Congress Control Number 2002106553

Additional copies of this report are available for sale from the National Academy Press, 2101 Constitution Avenue, N.W., Box 285, Washington, D.C. 20055. Call (800) 624-6242 or (202) 334-3313 (in the Washington metropolitan area), or visit the NAP's home page at **www.nap.edu**. The full text of this report is available at **www.nap.edu**.

For more information about the Institute of Medicine, visit the IOM home page at: **www.iom.edu**.

Copyright 2002 by the National Academy of Sciences. All rights reserved.

Printed in the United States of America.

The serpent has been a symbol of long life, healing, and knowledge among almost all cultures and religions since the beginning of recorded history. The serpent adopted as a logotype by the Institute of Medicine is a relief carving from ancient Greece, now held by the Staatliche Museen in Berlin.

*"Knowing is not enough; we must apply.
Willing is not enough; we must do."*
—Goethe

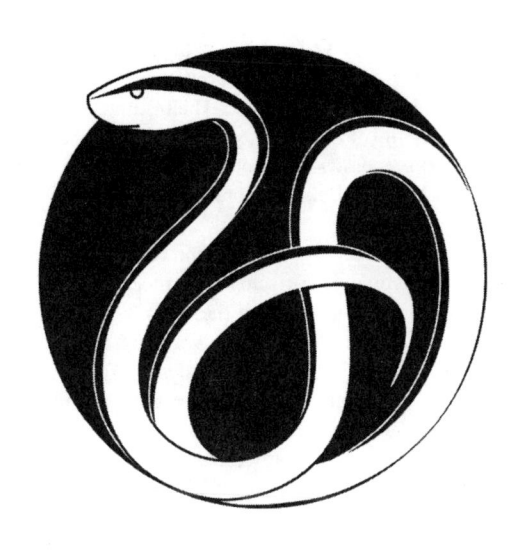

INSTITUTE OF MEDICINE

Shaping the Future for Health

THE NATIONAL ACADEMIES

National Academy of Sciences
National Academy of Engineering
Institute of Medicine
National Research Council

The **National Academy of Sciences** is a private, nonprofit, self-perpetuating society of distinguished scholars engaged in scientific and engineering research, dedicated to the furtherance of science and technology and to their use for the general welfare. Upon the authority of the charter granted to it by the Congress in 1863, the Academy has a mandate that requires it to advise the federal government on scientific and technical matters. Dr. Bruce M. Alberts is president of the National Academy of Sciences.

The **National Academy of Engineering** was established in 1964, under the charter of the National Academy of Sciences, as a parallel organization of outstanding engineers. It is autonomous in its administration and in the selection of its members, sharing with the National Academy of Sciences the responsibility for advising the federal government. The National Academy of Engineering also sponsors engineering programs aimed at meeting national needs, encourages education and research, and recognizes the superior achievements of engineers. Dr. Wm. A. Wulf is president of the National Academy of Engineering.

The **Institute of Medicine** was established in 1970 by the National Academy of Sciences to secure the services of eminent members of appropriate professions in the examination of policy matters pertaining to the health of the public. The Institute acts under the responsibility given to the National Academy of Sciences by its congressional charter to be an adviser to the federal government and, upon its own initiative, to identify issues of medical care, research, and education. Dr. Kenneth I. Shine is president of the Institute of Medicine.

The **National Research Council** was organized by the National Academy of Sciences in 1916 to associate the broad community of science and technology with the Academy's purposes of furthering knowledge and advising the federal government. Functioning in accordance with general policies determined by the Academy, the Council has become the principal operating agency of both the National Academy of Sciences and the National Academy of Engineering in providing services to the government, the public, and the scientific and engineering communities. The Council is administered jointly by both Academies and the Institute of Medicine. Dr. Bruce M. Alberts and Dr. Wm. A. Wulf are chairman and vice chairman, respectively, of the National Research Council.

CLINICAL RESEARCH ROUNDTABLE

WILLIAM GERBERDING, (*Co-chair*), President Emeritus, University of Washington, Seattle, Washington

ENRIQUETA BOND, (*Co-chair*) President, Burroughs Wellcome Fund, Research Triangle Park, North Carolina

TOM BEAUCHAMP, Professor of Philosophy and Senior Research Scholar, Kennedy Institute of Ethics, Georgetown University, Washington, D.C.

VERONICA CATANESE, Associate Dean, New York University School of Medicine, Director of Development, American Federation for Medical Research Foundation, New York, New York

FRANCIS CHESLEY, Director, Office of Research, Review, Education and Policy, Agency for Healthcare Research and Quality, Rockville, Maryland

WILLIAM F. CROWLEY, JR., Professor of Medicine, Harvard University, Director of Clinical Research, Massachusetts General Hospital, Boston, Massachusetts

ADRIAN DOBS, Professor of Medicine, Director, Clinical Research Unit, Johns Hopkins University School of Medicine, Baltimore, Maryland

JOHN FEUSSNER, Chief Research and Development Officer, Department of Veterans Affairs, Washington, D.C.

MYRON GENEL, Associate Dean, Office of Government and Community Affairs, Yale University School of Medicine, New Haven, Connecticut

KENNETH GETZ, President/Publisher, CenterWatch, Boston, Massachusetts

JACK GREBB, Senior Vice President, Johnson & Johnson, Global CNS/ Analgesia Clinical Research and Development, Janssen Research Foundation, Titusville, New Jersey

LAWRENCE GREEN, Director, Office of Extramural Prevention Research, Centers for Disease Control and Prevention, Atlanta, Georgia

STEPHEN KATZ, Director, National Institute of Arthritis and Musculoskeletal and Skin Diseases, Chief, Dermatology Branch, National Cancer Institute, Bethesda, Maryland

ALLAN M. KORN, Senior Vice President, Chief Medical Officer, Blue Cross Blue Shield Association, Chicago, Illinois

DAVID KORN, Senior Vice President for Biomedical and Health Sciences Research, Association of American Medical Colleges, Washington, D.C.

ELAINE L. LARSON, Professor of Pharmaceutical and Therapeutic Research, Columbia University School of Nursing, New York, New York

E. ALBERT REECE, Vice Chancellor and Dean, University of Arkansas College of Medicine, Little Rock, Arkansas

DAVID L. RIMOIN, Chairman of Pediatrics and Director, Medical Genetics-Birth Defects Center Cedars-Sinai Medical Center, Los Angeles, California

PATRICIA SALBER, Medical Director for Managed Care Health Care Initiative, General Motors Co., The Permanente Company, Larkspur, California
LEWIS SANDY, Executive Vice President, Robert Woods Johnson Foundation, Princeton, New Jersey
DAVID SCHEINBERG, Doris Duke Clinical Science Professor Chief, Leukemia Service, Memorial Sloan-Kettering Cancer, New York, New York
BERNARD SCHWETZ, Acting Deputy Commissioner and Senior Advisor for Science, Food and Drug Administration, Rockville, Maryland
LOUIS SHERWOOD, Senior Vice President for Medical and Scientific Affairs, Merck and Co., West Point, Pennsylvania
LANA SKIRBOLL, Director, Office of Science Policy, National Institutes of Health, Rockville, Maryland
HAROLD SLAVKIN, Dean, G. Donald and Marian James Montgomery Professor of Dentistry, School of Dentistry, University of Southern California, Los Angeles, California
SEAN TUNIS, Director, Coverage and Analysis Group, Office of Clinical Standards and Quality Centers for Medicare and Medicaid Services
MYRL WEINBERG, President, National Health Council, Washington, D.C.
MICHAEL J. WELCH, Co-Director, Division of Radiological Sciences, The Edward Mallincrodt Institute of Radiology, Washington University School of Medicine, St. Louis, Missouri

Liaisons to the Clinical Research Roundtable

STEVEN PAUL, Group Vice President, Lilly Research Laboratories, Eli Lilly and Company, Lilly Corporate Center
HUGH TILSON, Senior Advisor to the Dean, School of Public Health, University of North Carolina
MARY WOOLLEY, President, Research!America

Study Staff

ALEX OMMAYA, Study Director
ANDREA KALFOGLOU, Program Officer
VANESSA WALKER, Research Assistant
PERRY LUKSIN, Senior Project Assistant

Division Staff

ANDREW POPE, Division Director
ALDEN CHANG, Administrative Assistant
CARLOS GABRIEL, Financial Associate

LAURIE YELLE, Consultant

REVIEWERS

This report has been reviewed in draft form by individuals chosen for their diverse perspectives and technical expertise, in accordance with procedures approved by the NRC's Report Review Committee. The purpose of this independent review is to provide candid and critical comments that will assist the institution in making its published report as sound as possible and to ensure that the report meets institutional standards for objectivity, evidence, and responsiveness to the study charge. The review comments and draft manuscript remain confidential to protect the integrity of the deliberative process. We wish to thank the following individuals for their review of this report:

Edward Campion, M.D., New England Journal of Medicine
Carolyn Clancy, M.D., Agency for Healthcare Research and Quality (AHRQ)
Michael R. McGarvey, M.D., Chief Medical Officer BCBSNJ, Retired

Although the reviewers listed above have provided many constructive comments and suggestions, they were not asked to endorse the conclusions nor did they see the final draft of the report before its release. The review of this report was overseen by Mel Worth, Scholar-in-Residence, Institute of Medicine, who was responsible for making certain that an independent examination of this report was carried out in accordance with institutional procedures and that all review comments were carefully considered. Responsibility for the final content of this report rests entirely with the authoring committee and the institution.

Foreword

Enriqueta Bond, Ph.D.
*Liaison, Institute of Medicine
President, Burroughs Wellcome Fund
Research Triangle Park, North Carolina*

The Clinical Research Roundtable was convened by the Institute of Medicine in early 2000. Since then the roundtable has discussed many issues relevant to clinical research and has sponsored several symposia, the proceedings for which are available on its website www.iom.edu/crr. The roundtable brings together individuals from the academic health community, federal agencies sponsoring and regulating clinical research, private-sector sponsors of clinical research, foundations, public- and private-sector insurance programs, health plans and insurance companies, corporate purchasers of health care, and representatives of patient interests. Their mission is to discuss the challenges facing the Clinical Research Enterprise and the approaches that might be adapted to create a more supportive and efficient environment for the conduct of a broad agenda of high-quality clinical research to benefit the American public.

The roundtable provides a forum and sponsors workshops for discussion of approaches to resolving both acute and long-term issues affecting clinical research. It strives to enhance mutual understanding of clinical research between the scientific community and the general public, while improving the public's understanding of and participation in clinical studies.

Some issues germane to the development and continued vitality of clinical research include workforce career development in clinical research across the health professions; the linkage between discoveries in basic science and their application to improved patient care; the essential coordination of clinical research within and between research entities and disciplines; the ability of academic health centers to conduct clinical research and training; the broad participation of health professionals in clinical research across all practice settings and emerging health care systems; the timely incorporation into clinical practice of new research findings and findings on health outcomes; and the availability of financial and other data to monitor and assess the different components of patient- and population-based health research.

The Clinical Research Roundtable was created to provide a place where a very complicated set of actors, who are all very important to the Clinical Research Enterprise, could begin to talk to one another and gain a better understanding of each others' perspectives. The workshop has well launched us on that course. Many significant follow-up activities were exposed during the workshop that will allow us to continue to better identify and describe how to advance the Clinical Research Enterprise in ways that will greatly improve patient health. The ideas presented in this summary are exciting and display a great openness of the payer-purchaser community and a variety of efforts under way to the challenges that arose during the workshop.

This workshop focused specifically on what purchasers (employers) and payers (insurance companies) want from the Clinical Research Enterprise, what their role is with respect to the enterprise, and what they can contribute to it. Since its inception the Clinical Research Roundtable has been working to define the dimension and size of the Clinical Research Enterprise. We have identified how large and how fragmented the enterprise is, and we have determined that the advancement of the nation's health depends critically on all the pieces working together in a much better way than they do now and on our gaining better understanding of each other's roles.

The workshop explored the following questions with the purchasers and payers: What do purchasers and payers need from the Clinical Research Enterprise? How have current efforts in clinical research met your needs? What steps are necessary to improve the Clinical Research Enterprise? What are your top priorities for clinical research? Who should fund research studies? What are purchasers and payers willing to contribute to the Clinical Research Enterprise? Can you point to effective partnerships that have produced worthwhile results from the purchaser and payer perspectives? What are the most effective methods for addressing questions of interest for purchasers and payers?

The agenda of the workshop, as reflected in the summaries of the workshop presentations contained in this report, was organized to elicit the responses to these questions first from the perspective of purchasers (employers), then from the perspective of payers (health plans and insurance companies), and finally from the perspective of stakeholders (voluntary health associations and researchers). In the final session of the workshop, opportunities and challenges in the Clinical Research Enterprise were discussed from the perspective of all participants in the enterprise, including consumers. Although speakers expressed many diverse points of view during the workshop, all recognized the opportunity for health care purchasers, payers, researchers, and other stakeholders to work collaboratively, as part of the Clinical Research Enterprise, to meet the many challenges in this country's health care.

Contents

FOREWORD ix

WORKSHOP SUMMARY 1

INTRODUCTION TO THE WORKSHOP 5

1 THE ROLE OF PURCHASERS IN THE CLINICAL RESEARCH ENTERPRISE 9
Introduction, 9
What Purchasers Need from the Clinical Research Enterprise, 9
Pharmaceutical Costs and Value for Purchasers, 14
Translational Blocks, 16
Challenges for Purchasers in the Clinical Research Enterprise, 18
Proposal for a National Clinical Research Enterprise
  Coordinating Activity, 21
The Importance of Prevention Research, 22
Consumer Involvement, 24
Publication of a Research Priorities Proposal, 25
Summary, 26

2 THE ROLE OF PAYERS IN THE CLINICAL RESEARCH ENTERPRISE 29
Introduction, 29
What Payers Need from the Clinical Research Enterprise, 30
What Payers Are Willing to Contribute to the Clinical Research Enterprise, 37
Research Priorities and Priority Setting for Payers, 40
Translational Blocks, 43
Consumer Demand, 47
Patient Participation in Clinical Research, 48
Summary, 48

3 THE ROLE OF OTHER STAKEHOLDERS IN THE CLINICAL RESEARCH ENTERPRISE 51
Introduction, 51
The Role of Voluntary Health Associations in the Clinical Research Enterprise, 52
Priority Setting in Basic and Clinical Research, 56
Priority Setting in Health Services Research, 58
Health Services Research in Voluntary Health Associations, 61
The Role of the Device Industry in the Clinical Research Enterprise, 63
The Role of the Agency for Healthcare Research and Quality in the Clinical Research Enterprise, 65
Translational Blocks and Practice Guidelines, 66
Summary, 68

4 OPPORTUNITIES AND CHALLENGES IN THE CLINICAL RESEARCH ENTERPRISE 70
Introduction, 70
Outcomes Research and Disease Management, 71
Integrated Patient-Centered Care, 75
Research Priorities in Pharmaceutical Companies, 75
Summary, 80

SUGGESTED READINGS　　　　　　　　　　　　　　　　82

APPENDIX I: Speaker Biographies　　　　　　　　　　　　83

APPENDIX II Speaker's Company Profiles　　　　　　　　90

APPENDIX III: Purchaser Payer Background Information　94

APPENDIX IV: Workshop Agenda 97

APPENDIX V: Definitions of Clinical Research and Components of the
  Enterprise 101
    Definition of Clinical Research, 101
    Major Components of the Clinical Research Enterprise, 101

APPENDIX VI: Registered Workshop Participants 103

Workshop Summary

The goal of the workshop that is the topic of this summary report, *The Role of Purchasers and Payers in the Clinical Research Enterprise,* was to examine how purchasers and payers interact with the various components of the Clinical Research Enterprise and to understand their perspective on what the vision of the enterprise should be. Representatives from purchaser organizations (employers), payer organizations (health plans and insurance companies), and other stakeholder organizations (voluntary health associations, researchers, research organizations, and the technology community) came together to explore the following questions: What do purchasers and payers need from the Clinical Research Enterprise? How have current efforts in clinical research met their needs? What are purchasers, payers, and other stakeholders willing to contribute to the enterprise? The workshop integrated the diverse views of the stakeholders and created a lively dialogue among the participants. Clinical research is defined broadly in this research, encompassing all patient oriented research, health services research, epidemiology, outcomes, and behavior research (see Appendix V). The language presented in this respect should not be viewed as an endorsement by the Clinical Research Roundtable or the Institute of Medicine of future action that is needed, but rather as an effort to synthesize the various perspectives presented.

The introductory presentation by the co-chairs of the workshop (Sean Tunis, M.D., of the Centers of Medicare and Medicaid Services, and Allan Korn, M.D., of the Blue Cross and Blue Shield Association) set the tone by emphasizing how quality of care depends on the quality of information underlying health care decisions. The speakers then postulated that the Clinical Research Enterprise currently does not produce an adequate volume or quality of information to support policy decision making at various levels—from employers, physician groups, government health programs, and health plans, to the ultimate end users, the consumers. Against this background, speakers from purchaser, payer, and other stakeholder organizations laid out a mosaic of views.

In the first session, *The Role of Purchasers in the Clinical Research Enterprise,* representatives of large employers and business organizations (General Motors Corporation, United Parcel Service, the National Business Coalition on Health, Verizon, the Washington Business Group on Health, Marriott International, and William M. Mercer Inc.) responded by describing what they need from the Clinical Research Enterprise. Speakers agreed that purchasers need the enterprise to provide them with knowledge of new technological innovations and treatments that have been proven effective through evidence from well-designed, well-executed, unbiased studies. They stated their need to understand why clinical practices vary widely and why agreed-upon practices are not uniformly performed, and they requested help in reducing this variation. They expressed their willingness to pay for quality in health care, but noted that they need to know what they will receive for their investment, either in the short-term or the long-term.

Purchasers recognized a trend toward a consumer-driven health care system in this country, and they acknowledged the important contribution that they can make in preventive health by educating their members and encouraging healthy lifestyle behaviors. They expressed interest in contributing to a national fund that would be used to examine research questions of national significance that are not currently being addressed, but they reiterated that they would need to know what the return would be for their investment. Finally, they considered the possibility of joining with payers to compile and publish a list of top-priority clinical research projects.

In the second session, *The Role of Payers in the Clinical Research Enterprise,* speakers from four health plans (Wellmark, HealthPartners, United Healthgroup, and Aetna U.S. Healthcare) and a representative from the American Association of Health Plans revisited many themes brought out in the purchaser session. They emphasized their need to understand what is effective and what is not in the care of patients, the prevention of disease, and the promotion of health. They discussed the need for full disclosure of information regarding research funding to the public, potential research participants, and other stakeholders. They acknowledged the need to know how to provide safer care and eliminate errors to keep members free from harm. They requested guidance on how to transform the culture of medical practice from a profession-centered, individual activity into a patient-centered, team effort. They wished for more insight into population-based community methods of improving individual and community health, and they asked for help in eliminating barriers to the delivery of interventions for behavioral change.

Payers acknowledged that the Clinical Research Enterprise provides innovations that improve care, prevent illness, and promote health. They recognized that the enterprise questions existing practice and helps eliminate ineffective and even harmful practices. They expressed their willingness to encourage dissemination of medical technologies of proven safety and effectively and to support the implementation of evidence-based guidelines and consensus statements in clinical practice. Further, they emphasized the important role that they play in imparting health information to their members through health education programs and encouraging healthy behaviors.

The third session, *The Role of Other Stakeholders in the Clinical Research Enterprise,* brought together representatives from voluntary health organizations (the American Cancer Society and the American Diabetes Association), researchers, the medical technology community (the Medical Technology Leadership Forum), and the Agency for Healthcare Research and Quality to discuss their contributions to the Clinical Research Enterprise and what they need from it to better promote health and health care. Speakers from the American Cancer Society and the American Diabetes Association described the contributions of their organizations to the Clinical Research Enterprise, which included participating in and funding clinical research, translating research into clinical practice, aiding in the creation of clinical guidelines, and advocating for funding and high-quality care for every patient. They acknowledged their special role in educating professionals, patients, and the public in health care and prevention.

Representatives of the academic research institutions discussed the deficiencies in the current research structure and called for a new type of research, evaluative research, that requires setting priorities for health care and working cooperatively to conduct research that is closely aligned with those priorities. They affirmed that researchers can assist the progress of the Clinical Research Enterprise by working with purchasers and payers to evaluate the impact of collaborative programs and interventions. A speaker from the medical technology community emphasized the unique characteristics of the medical device industry, such as short product life cycles and high clinical trial costs per unit, and called for assistance from the Clinical Research Enterprise in evaluating new technology. A representative of the Agency for Healthcare Research and Quality described its mission, which is to support and conduct research that will improve health outcomes, quality of care, and cost and utilization of health care services. Participants in this session also identified the need for a paradigm shift away from the current individual investigator-driven research toward research based on wide collaboration and teamwork.

The goal of the final session of the workshop, *Opportunities and Challenges in the Clinical Research Enterprise,* was to explore opportunities for new approaches to research and patient care and examine challenges associated with research funding. These topics engendered discussion by participants representing a wide range of stakeholder interests. A representative from Merck and Company presented an example of outcomes research, which examines the consequences of medical treatment in terms of what is important to those being treated and leads to disease management. During the ensuing discussion an initiative called integrated patient-centered care, which goes beyond disease management by considering the whole person, was described. A lively discussion centered around the issue of conflict of interest in industry-funded research.

In conclusion, prevailing themes throughout the workshop were the need for research to determine what does and does not work in treatment, diagnosis, and prevention; the need to translate basic science research into clinical recommendations, and clinical guidelines into consistently practiced best evidence-based care; and the need to transform the professional health care culture into a team effort. Participants recognized the trend toward a consumer-driven health care system, and they affirmed their commitment to the public good. They came away from the workshop with a clearer understanding of each others' views and a commitment to search for unique solutions to the nation's health care questions and to work together to apply them.

Introduction to the Workshop

Sean Tunis, M.D., M.Sc.
Workshop Co-Chair
Director, Coverage and Analysis Group
Office of Clinical Standards and Quality
Centers for Medicare and Medicaid Services
and
Allan Korn, M.D.
Workshop Co-Chair
Senior Vice President and Chief Medical Office
Blue Cross Blue Shield Association

(Presented by Sean Tunis)

The topic of this workshop, *The Role of Purchasers and Payers in the Clinical Research Enterprise,* is critical to the quality of patient care, in the sense that the quality of care depends on the quality of information underlying health care decisions. Without high-quality empirical information to support decision making in health policy and clinical care, the quality of patient care cannot possibly be improved. The role of the Clinical Research Enterprise itself is underemphasized and under-highlighted in the quality-of-care discussion. Little consensus exists as to what role purchasers and payers should play in the Clinical Research Enterprise and how that role can be improved. The Clinical Research Roundtable hopes to make headway in addressing these issues through this workshop.

> Without high-quality empirical information to support decision making in health policy and clinical care, the quality of patient care cannot possibly be improved.
>
> —*Sean Tunis*

The Clinical Research Enterprise is a broadly defined term that includes a wide spectrum of research and its applications—from the beginnings of human-oriented practical bench-top research and its application to patient care, to clinical epidemiology, health services research, and outcomes research. Even further along the spectrum is the incorporation of these findings into health care in the community. The view of Sean Tunis of the Centers for Medicare and Medicaid Services and Allan Korn of the Blue Cross Blue Shield Association, as self-described evidence-based decision makers in large insurance organizations, is that, as currently configured, the Clinical Research Enterprise does not produce

> The Clinical Research Enterprise does not produce an adequate volume or quality of information to support policy decision making at a number of different levels—hospitals; physician groups; and large organizational levels such as the Medicare program and health insurance companies.
>
> —Sean Tunis

an adequate volume or quality of information to support policy decision making at a number of different levels—hospitals; physician groups; and large organizational levels such as the Medicare program and health insurance companies.

Groups poorly served by the output of the Clinical Research Enterprise are consumers, clinicians, payers, purchasers, and health care policy makers—a fairly large and important group of end users of research. Particularly poorly served are clinicians, who need high-quality information that speaks to the practical questions that they encounter in day-to-day patient care, and consumers, who count on the quality of evidence available to them to properly inform them in making health care decisions.

For example, many women have had to make personal decisions about the use of hormone replacement therapy for the prevention of osteoporosis and its complications. For years, that decision was driven largely by the purported impact of hormone replacement therapy on cardiovascular disease, because that health outcome far outweighed any impact on osteoporosis risk in terms of magnitude of morbidity. Many years of epidemiologic and observational studies suggested that hormone replacement therapy was beneficial in terms of cardiovascular disease. However, well-designed prospective clinical trials recently demonstrated that the benefit was either nonexistent or extremely small.

The example shows that personal decisions that patients and physicians make about health care depend critically on the quality and integrity of the information produced by the Clinical Research Enterprise. If the enterprise is not producing an adequate number of studies, of adequate reliability, to properly inform those decisions, it is failing an important group of users. That perception underlies the urgency and importance of making some headway in this workshop, identifying follow-up activities, and determining how the Clinical Research Enterprise can be more productive in the area of studies that support this kind of decision making.

When government and private health insurers try to develop coverage policy in an evidence-based fashion—for instance, deciding which new and old technologies to pay for—the evidence is often lacking. Increasingly, large systematic reviews of published clinical literature are commissioned on the most commonly used technologies, and they generally reveal that the research available is inadequate to support evidence-based decision making. For example, it is almost impossible to develop sensible evidence-based coverage policy on the use of virtually any type of new wound care therapy on patients with pressure ulcers. We just do not know whether air fluidized beds, electrical stimulation, hyperbaric oxygen, or any number of other things do anything to speed the healing of pressure ulcers. Yet we spend tens of millions of dollars and much patient and caregiver time on those sorts of interventions. In this area the Clinical Research Enterprise is unaccountably silent. This problem grows more acute as the pace of medical innovation increases. Although huge sums of money are invested in the development of promising new technologies, a matching investment in the value of the clinical utility of new innovations is lacking. Thus, potentially useful innovations are put into the marketplace, at a faster and faster rate, yet there is no matched effort to determine how those innovations appropriately fit into the armamentarium of clinical care.

> Thus, potentially useful innovations are put into the marketplace, at a faster and faster rate, partially the result of doubling the budget of the National Institutes of Health; yet there is no matched effort to determine how those innovations appropriately fit into the armamentarium of clinical care.
>
> —Allan Korn

Payers, certainly, but also all other end users, such as purchasers and consumers, must be much more active participants in the Clinical Research Enterprise. They must participate in setting priorities for clinical research, assisting in the design of clinical research, and probably participating to a much greater degree in its funding. Certain stakeholders also need to become involved in recruiting patients into clinical research to answer important research questions. Unless these end users become active participants in every phase of the Clinical Research Enterprise, it will not change dramatically to better serve their needs.

Similarly, the Clinical Research Enterprise must look to the end users much more as true partners in the enterprise rather than as "deep pockets" to provide additional funding for clinical research. What is needed is not more support for the clinical research that is already being done, but rather support for a different kind of clinical research. Some examples of this new type of research already exist. The Veterans Administration performs applied, practical clinical research that supports decision making. Another program, the Centers for Education and Research on Therapeutics (CERT) funded through the Food and Drug Administration (FDA) and the Agency for Healthcare Research and Quality (AHRQ), has begun a number of studies to fill the gaps in what physicians and patients need to know to support decision making.

> Similarly, the Clinical Research Enterprise must look to the end users much more as true partners in the enterprise than as "deep pockets" to provide additional funding for clinical research.
>
> —Sean Tunis

The research community must recognize that a move to this new type of research leads down a long, difficult road and marks a serious shift in the emphasis of the Clinical Research Enterprise that poses huge challenges in methodology and infrastructure. Researchers need to be properly trained in this new type of clinical research, or in research that answers slightly different questions. Some of this shift in emphasis is being driven unilaterally by purchasers and payers who are increasingly taking a more active role. The goal can be accomplished by the payer-purchaser community coming together and bringing its funds and resources to bear on this movement in a new direction. It can be best achieved, however, when all components of the enterprise cooperate with each other.

> The research community must recognize that a move to this new type of research leads down a long, difficult road and marks a serious shift in the emphasis of the Clinical Research Enterprise that poses huge challenges in methodology and infrastructure.
>
> —Sean Tunis

1

The Role of Purchasers in the Clinical Research Enterprise

INTRODUCTION

Patricia R. Salber, M.D., M.B.A.
Medical Director, Managed Care, Health Care Initiatives
General Motors Corporation in conjunction with The Permanente Company

This part of the workshop deals with the perspective of private purchasers, a perspective not often included in in-depth discussions related to clinical research. The goal is to understand how the Clinical Research Enterprise can better serve purchasers as they strive to provide high-quality, affordable health care benefits to employees, retirees, and dependents. During this session, purchasers will elucidate what they need from the Clinical Research Enterprise and outline their contributions to it. They will also speak about the challenges they face in translating research into practice. Translational blocks are encountered on the road from basic science to improved health and health care for individuals. The first and most familiar block is in the translation of basic science into clinically meaningful recommendations. The second translational block is in turning those recommendations into action. The ways in which purchasers are affected by both of these blocks will be discussed. Finally, consumer involvement in the Clinical Research Enterprise and its impact on purchasers will be explored.

WHAT PURCHASERS NEED FROM THE CLINICAL RESEARCH ENTERPRISE

Dale Whitney
Corporate Health and Welfare Manager
United Parcel Service

United Parcel Service (UPS) invests roughly $1.6 billion for health care coverage for its employees, retirees, and their families. Next year, that investment will increase by about 10%. Whenever the Board of Directors and shareholders make an investment, particularly one that increases at this rate, they want to know what UPS will receive for the additional investment. Will the workforce be 10% healthier? Will customer satisfaction increase by 10%? Will the investment somehow add to the bottom line of the enterprise or add to the public good? Or will the additional dollars simply be spent with no return?

As we move toward a consumer-driven health care system, information must become available to the consumer, and not just to the purchaser or clinician. The information must support effective health care decision making at all levels of the system. A current concern is that treatment for the same clinical condition varies widely, raising several questions: If providers receive a similar education and read the same articles in the professional journals, why is there so much treatment variation within the system? Should employers provide coverage and benefits for all variations?

> Purchasers are looking for ways to promote and improve quality in providers. Although they are willing to change their contracts to support this goal, they have not yet found effective models.
>
> —Dale Whitney

It has been said that employers are not willing to pay for quality in health care, but this is not the case. Purchasers are willing to differentiate and pay more for quality care because high-quality care saves money in the long run by improving satisfaction and performance in our workforce. Purchasers are looking for ways to promote and improve quality in providers. Although they are willing to change their contracts to support this goal, they have not yet found effective models.

Gregg Lehman, Ph.D.
President and Corporate Executive Officer
National Business Coalition on Health

The National Business Coalition on Health (NBCH), on behalf of its nearly 90 employer-led coalitions nationwide and their 8,000 employers and approximately 30 million covered lives, recognize the outstanding clinical research that has taken place to date. Therapeutic investigations, especially in the area of pharmaceutical products, have made the U.S.A. the leader in the development of new drugs and medical devices. Many of these products have resulted in a healthier and more productive workforce for purchasers. We are pleased that current therapeutic interventions are largely focused on the those conditions identified in the Institute of Medicine report *Crossing the Quality Chasm: A New Health System for the 21st Century* (Committee on Quality of Health Care in America, Institute of Medicine, 2001) that account for about 80% of health care spending

These conditions represent not only large direct health care expense but also indirect costs in terms of absenteeism and lost productivity that often outweigh the direct expense. Unfortunately, purchasers are without tools to measure the impact of both new and current interventions on the productivity of their workforce.

The state-of-the-art work in the field of epidemiology has broadened our knowledge of the patterns of disease within subsets of the population as well as across the population. Although health services and outcomes research have made an effort to better understand the "real world" of health care, much more needs to be done. The NBCH member coalitions' purchasers are committed to purchasing health care for their employees, dependents, and retirees based on value—high quality at an appropriate price. Yet research-based, standardized metrics to evaluate most of the dimensions of providers' and hospitals' performance are lacking. Nor has research identified optimal approaches for the dissemination of performance information to purchasers in support of their purchasing efforts.

Health services research has also not fully addressed the translation of research into practice. For example, evidence-based medical guidelines, founded on significant clinical research, have been developed for many of the conditions identified in the IOM report *Crossing the Quality Chasm: A New Health System for the 21st Century* (2001). Yet health services researchers and others have found that physicians and other health care providers frequently do not follow such guidelines. Purchasers, and the country's health care system as a whole, would greatly benefit from health services research that would help to define mechanisms by which purchasers, plans, and payers could encourage not merely the broad adoption of evidence-based clinical guidelines, but also their integration into the day-to-day delivery of health care services. We know that purchasers can play an integral role in "integrating research into practice" through contracting methodology as well as integrating the work of the Leapfrog group in implementing research-based patient safety standards.

> The country's health care system as a whole, would greatly benefit from health services research that would help to define mechanisms by which purchasers, plans, and payers could encourage not merely the broad adoption of evidence-based clinical guidelines, but also their integration into the day-to-day delivery of health care services.
>
> —Gregg Lehman

Research in the area of prevention and health promotion has yielded standardized clinical guidelines, which offer significant opportunities to improve the health of the current U.S. population. Unfortunately, these preventative services are often not received, even when a service is a covered benefit under the purchaser's health plan. As an example, consider the variation in the following preventative services:

- Up-to-date Pap smear testing from 70% to 93%
- Cholesterol screening from 45% to 88%
- Tobacco cessation advice from 20% to 77% (Solbert et al., 2001)

Purchasers would greatly benefit from health services research that aids in the understanding of the reasons for variation in receipt of preventative services as well as solutions to reduce the variation. For example, could changes in benefit design (e.g., change in co-pay) increase the receipt of preventative services? Or would time off from work to obtain needed services increase the percentage of employees that receive such services?

NBCH coalitions and the purchasers that they represent are committed to value-based purchasing. As such they would benefit from increased health services research in the following areas:

- Development of metrics that would differentiate physician, hospital, and other health care provider performance
- Identification of incentive systems that would "reward" optimal provider practice, and similarly, identification of incentive systems that would encourage employees to proactively manage their own health and to seek care (preventative, episodic, and chronic) from top-performing providers
- Creation of metrics to quantify the impact on worker productivity of high-quality health care that is delivered in accordance with evidence-based clinical guidelines.

> Many chief financial officers want a business case to be made for the cost of quality improvement programs.
>
> —Gregg Lehman

Many chief financial officers want a business case to be made for the cost of quality improvement programs, i.e., a return on investment for paying for quality. Simply put, if outcomes associated with following guidelines can be measured and their impact in terms of dollars translated, the business case will be made. Purchasers are a long way from making that case. If a business case is made, a rapid realignment of incentives would follow.

Bruce Taylor
Director of National Health Care and Policy Plans
Verizon

Dissemination of clinical information that is known to be effective is an important issue in improving the health care system. Best-practice clinical information and treatment plans should be in the hands of providers, purchasers, and consumers. For example, there is much concern about diabetes, heart disease, and other conditions that drive up health care costs. In tomorrow's health care environment, the whole discussion could change dramatically when the prospects of the genome project are considered. Almost 'overnight' the focus could change from providing treatment to maintaining health and preventing disease.

A key issue to patients and purchasers is "value," which raises many questions: What do purchasers get for the additional expenditure involved? What value does the consumer receive, and what does the payer receive? Purchasers have tried many approaches to obtain quality care for their employees. The complaints often heard are that purchasers are not paying enough, with the reasoning that increased reimbursement for medical services will translate to better or higher quality care. And, many purchasers currently negotiate price rather than quality.

> Purchasers are now negotiating price rather than quality. The point is that there are employers who are trying to pay for quality.
>
> —Bruce Taylor

Changing the cost paradigm is not easy. However, it is possible if clinical, quality, and cost goals are aligned. For example, several large employers recently expressed their willingness to pay more—in this case bonuses—to hospitals that were able to meet two Leapfrog safety standards for improving patient care. The point is that there are employers who are trying to pay for quality. Purchasers are eager to consider any ideas regarding how to push the agenda forward. It is known that, like manufacturing, improving the quality drives costs down while improving customer satisfaction.

Helen Darling
President
Washington Business Group on Health

As seen in the latest debate about the utility of mammography guidelines, fundamental research performed years ago was often not conducted in a way that allowed answers to basic questions. Today purchasers want new technologies and treatments to have been proven efficacious based on high standards of clinical empirical evidence. This type of research is not available in many cases. Studies should be well designed, well executed, and published in peer-reviewed journals. Regrettably, the percentage of studies meeting these criteria is shockingly low.

> Studies should be well designed and well executed, and results should be published in peer-reviewed journals. Regrettably, the percentage of studies meeting these criteria is shockingly low.
>
> —Helen Darling

Ideally, results will be based on the gold standard—randomized controlled clinical trials—but this standard cannot always be met, either because the number of cases is small or because the treatment is already in practice. If it is not possible to meet the gold standard, then we should at least meet the best standards possible. Everyone involved in health care and coverage should be appropriately skeptical of claims in the absence of solid evidence. Developers of new technologies or treatments tend to be enthusiastic, and that is laudable. It should be recognized, however, that the drive and enthusiasm that make it possible for them to develop these treatments sometimes do affect their judgment and their assertions.

To make matters worse, media reporting of new therapies often focuses on benefits with almost no attention given to harmful effects. Politicians, narrow special interests, and the courts all become involved and sometimes drive decisions that are fundamentally wrong and downright harmful. The result is not only harm but also lost opportunities.

This nation has a $1.5 trillion health care industry. Many purchasers feel this amount is ample for health care in general. To find budgetary room for new technology and new treatments that are effective—that make a real difference in health and productivity—ineffective or less-than-effective technology must be driven out. Yet this is almost never done. In the United States new technology is often layered on the old. Both new and old are continued, partly because evidence is lacking.

The Clinical Research Enterprise provides more innovation, more new technology, and more new drugs than any enterprise in the world. Purchasers are more than willing to help disseminate information on best clinical practices and reward hospitals, physicians, and others who are willing to meet best-practice standards. For this to happen, providers themselves must agree on best practices. It is hard to make changes if clinicians are ambivalent about what constitutes best practices, either because they are unfamiliar with the evidence or because the evidence is not available.

Purchasers must do a better job of re-packaging health care information to make it accessible to consumers. Also, they need to know more about why agreed-upon practices are not performed by 100% of providers. Purchasers want providers to use evidence-based clinical guidelines. The important questions are, how do we identify those providers who follow the guidelines and obtain the outcomes that we are looking for, how do we pay for the high-quality care they provide, and what is the right amount to pay?

PHARMACEUTICAL COSTS AND VALUE FOR PURCHASERS
Patricia Salber, M.D., M.B.A.

An important issue for purchasers is pharmaceutical costs. At General Motors, these costs now exceed inpatient costs with respect to many of our health plans. In the current environment of escalating health care costs, payers are focusing much attention on drug expenditures. Sometimes their methods do not make the best sense clinically because they lack information needed to make better decisions. In this regard, more head-to-head comparisons of the value of new versus existing therapeutic agents could help purchasers make more rational benefit design decisions.

Jill Berger
Corporate Health and Welfare Manager
Marriott International

Many purchasers are again experiencing double-digit inflation in medical costs, which is a large concern for Marriott. Marriott offers enrollment in 70 health maintenance organizations to its employees across the country. It also has a preferred provider organization that is managed to some degree. Marriott's business strategy will not allow us to go forward with double-digit increases without understanding where the dollars are going. An area of great concern is pharmaceutical costs. As with General Motors, those costs are beginning to exceed inpatient costs. This situation is of concern to Marriott because many new drugs being brought into the marketplace will be very expensive, and the company will be forced to make difficult decisions regarding coverage. Purchasers will need research to help them make those decisions.

No forum exists for assessing drug value in the U.S.A. today. Purchasers would like to see studies that include drug comparison, affordability, and safety. A number of stakeholders recently joined together to form RxValue Health. Consumers, providers, health plans, and employers are part of this effort. The members finance a great deal of the health care in the country, and their goal is to address the question of whether purchasers as well as their employees receive value in relation to the rapidly increasing pharmaceutical costs. The coalition's combined members represent the interests of 135 million Americans as it attempts to assess and secure value for the resources spent on pharmaceuticals. The coalition members would like independent governmental agencies to fund research to help evaluate which drugs provide good value. Members are concerned with new expensive branded drugs that provide no more value than current agents.

RxValue Health members want to use the answers to their questions to help inform policy makers as well as businesses and consumers. They advocate research in the following areas:

- Policy research to assess the market rules that impair open and effective competition
- Clinical research to differentiate new drugs from "improved" drugs or "me-too" drugs

- Economic research to assess the cost of proposals for patent and/or market exclusivity expansions
- Research on the costs of the delay of entry of generic pharmaceuticals to consumers and employers
- Unbiased drug studies not funded by the pharmaceutical industry
- Studies on the pediatric utilization of selections of drugs that receive pediatric-based exclusivity extensions (i.e., an additional six months of marketing exclusivity when the sponsor submits pediatric testing information relating to the use of the drug in the pediatric population)

Purchasers also need help in setting their plan design regarding what to pay for and when, and how to pay for it. For example, three-tier co-pays are currently popular. In fact, Marriott included them in all health plans this year. The impact of the three-tier formulary on appropriate drugs needs to be examined. Marriott wants to make sure that the tiers are structured so that all appropriate drugs are available on all the tiers.

TRANSLATIONAL BLOCKS

Jon Hautz, C.E.B.S.
Senior Consultant
William M. Mercer Inc.

> Do we put accurate information into the users' hands? Pick up any popular women's magazine and see how many surveys, research findings, or health recommendations are included. From month to month and year to year, startling conflicts can be found in the health information reported.
>
> —Jon Hautz

It is important for purchasers to consider the health care information that ultimately filters down to the user level. Tomorrow, employers may not be the ones who choose health plans for their employees. A trend in this country is to move that purchasing decision down to consumers—to inform them about available benefits and available funds (i.e., a defined medical spending/savings account) and let them spend these contributed dollars on whatever medical care they wish. End users must have the information that they need to make wise choices. Do we put accurate information into the users' hands? Pick up any popular women's magazine and see how many surveys, research findings, or health recommendations are included. From month to month and year to year, startling conflicts can be found in the health information reported. Difficulty in communicating to the end users what works in health care is a translational block. If the research is unfocused at the top level, the people who are the recipients of that research are going to be totally in the dark.

Gregg Lehman, Ph.D.

In 2001, the NBCH created the not-for-profit Clinical Performance Enhancement Center (CPEC). The mission of the CPEC is to provide a national setting and structure in which health care provider quality and effectiveness can be accurately evaluated at the clinical level and reported with the objectives of improving the health care provided to the general public regardless of payer, assisting providers in achieving best demonstrated practices, and making information available to further research into healthcare delivery.

The Lipid Project (a "Project to Enhance Compliance with National and Local Evidence-Based Cholesterol Guidelines") is the initial provider performance enhancement project of the CPEC. The project is funded by an unrestricted grant from AstraZeneca to the NBCH.

The goal of the multi-year project is to demonstrate, in an ambulatory care setting, a provider clinical performance reporting capability utilizing evidence-based medicine guidelines in a high-incidence, relatively low compliance and high risk condition (e.g., elevated cholesterol) and the applicability of expanding that capability to regional and/or national levels. The project is using two ambulatory settings for the study—a Philadelphia area provider site and a Baltimore area provider site. In January 2002, the lipid project will be expanded to a statewide initiative in Maryland and will expand purchaser involvement to the public sector.

> When purchasers find out what is working, they need to build this information into their contract methodology and give incentives not just to providers but also to employees so that they maintain compliance with these interventions.
>
> —Gregg Lehman

The CPEC lipid project demonstrates the effective partnership of purchasers, researchers, physicians and pharmaceutical manufacturers. The CPEC project also contains many of the facets of research that are important to purchasers. These elements include the evaluation of:

- Provider performance using evidence-based clinical guidelines
- Relative effectiveness of health plan interventions in changing physician practice patterns
- Impact of employee interventions in eliciting the desired behavior
- Potential mechanisms to support use of project data to support value-based purchasing

The important outcome of this project is guidance on realignment of incentives. When purchasers find out what is working, they need to build this information into their contract methodology and give incentives not just to providers but also to employees so that they maintain compliance with these interventions. Employers are very concerned about not only the direct cost of the drugs used to treat diseases but also the indirect costs associated with the disease states—how these conditions impact productivity and how they impact absenteeism, for example.

Dale Whitney

Research that has a real impact will involve the physician who actually sees 500 patients a month. Purchasers need to learn from such providers how they absorb research findings and apply them to their practice. This important piece is often overlooked. It is not surprising that providers have difficulty incorporating research findings into practice when health care guidelines and recommendations are constantly changing. Providers are expected to know these guidelines by rote, but why should this be so when technology is available? Technology needs to be brought into the mix so that providers have all relevant information at their fingertips, not just in their minds. There is just too much health care information today, and it changes too often for anyone to be expected to remember it all. Imagine if UPS tracked its packages in its employees' minds rather than by computer!

CHALLENGES FOR PURCHASERS IN THE CLINICAL RESEARCH ENTERPRISE

Patricia Salber, M.D., M.B.A

Purchasers seem to be "marching to a different drummer" than academic researchers because of the urgency of their need for answers to the questions that they face, particularly in light of double-digit inflation of health care costs in the context of an economic downturn. Effective partnerships are those that provide the flexibility to address both short-term and long-term needs, yet purchasers' short-term needs often cannot be met by the slow pace of the research process. To cite an example, General Motors spent three or four months putting together a grant proposal for funding the development of a return-on-investment methodology. The company waited another six or seven months for the public agency to hear whether it had been recommended for funding. Although the proposal did receive a high score and was recommended for funding, General Motors is now in its third month of waiting to hear whether that recommendation will translate into dollars. A one-year time frame before the research begins does not work well for purchasers. There needs to be a mechanism that will allow a faster track review for priority purchaser research issues.

Dale Whitney

One challenge to purchasers is the conflict of interest in funding research efforts. Several times a year a representative from a pharmaceutical company promotes drug-based disease management programs at UPS. It is difficult to evaluate a program in which most evidence for its utility is from studies funded by the pharmaceutical industry. UPS would like evidence from studies funded by sources that have no conflict of interest before trying out a program on its 750,000 beneficiaries.

Bruce Taylor

A particular challenge faced by purchasers is how to make what they spend for health care more valuable. Verizon tells its employees that there is no money tree. Rather, available resources are constantly reallocated. Similarly, the Clinical Research Enterprise needs to address how the $1.5 trillion available for health care can best be utilized for the benefit of not only today's patients but also tomorrow's.

The $1.5 trillion expended annually for health care in the U.S.A. certainly seems to be plenty of money. The number of dollars is unimportant. What is essential is the value received for that investment. In a discussion a few years ago between several employers, including Verizon, and the director of the National Institutes of Health, the employers recommended that research support ought to be broad-based, and that it should not come from any particular segment of society. Perhaps part of the general income tax should be used for this purpose. And, there should be a clear sense of the amount of support available for all levels of research.

Helen Darling

An important challenge is the proper evaluation of research. The Department of Health and Human Services used to earmark a certain amount of money for evaluation. As a consequence, much evaluation was performed that would

> As a nation, we need to earmark some portion of every health institution's budget that can only be spent on [evaluation research].
>
> —Helen Darling

not have been done otherwise. As a nation, we need to earmark some portion of every health institution's budget that can only be spent on this kind of application and translation. The amount should be reasonable, perhaps 5% of the budget. All members of the research community should pool their interests and desires and declare that the value will be gained if translation of health care information can be improved. Such an effort will help consumers, taxpayers, and purchasers, and it will help the Clinical Research Enterprise itself. Perhaps we could all work together toward that goal.

David Rimoin, M.D., Ph.D.
*Chairman of Pediatrics and Director of
Medical Genetics Birth Defects Center
Cedars Sinai Medical Center*

Genomics will pose new challenges for purchasers in coming years. Purchasers want good productivity indices and more value for their health care dollar; yet they are frustrated because the research studies coming out are nonuniform or ambiguous. In the future, studies will become even less uniform and more ambiguous because of the genome project.

Through pharmacogenomics, researchers are finding that individuals will vary tremendously in their response to a given pharmaceutical agent or treatment method based on their particular genetic predisposition. Finding out what works for a particular patient means allowing individuals to expose themselves genetically. First, there must be much better protection against genetic discrimination in insurance coverage and in the workplace. Genetic differences might affect job performance and absenteeism, and they might affect the cost of individual health care. Individuals must be examined as individuals to find out what is best for them in terms of health treatment, but we must also protect them from "pulling down their genes." In the end, results will be much better if people are treated as individuals genetically, but this effort will require a monetary investment and an understanding that there is not a uniform answer for everything.

Greg Lehman, Ph.D.

The area of pharmacogenomics is fascinating and also frightening to the employer community for the very reasons just mentioned. Targeted intervention for subgroups within disease states is a fascinating topic, but the costs and benefits are unknown. The area warrants in-depth study, and there are many unknowns for the employer community. If targeted interventions can produce a lasting effect, health care savings may be substantial.

PROPOSAL FOR A NATIONAL CLINICAL RESEARCH ENTERPRISE COORDINATING ACTIVITY

William Crowley, M.D.
*Professor of Medicine, Harvard University, and
Director of Clinical Research, Reproductive Endocrine Unit
Massachusetts General Hospital*

Purchasers, in aggregate, are unhappy about the rising costs of health care and the decreasing information on quality and variability in the implementation of practices, guidelines, and safety. Purchasers respond in some cases by jiggling the reimbursement level as the "carrot and stick" at the same time. Other efforts include conducting the applied studies mentioned above. The Clinical Research Roundtable has been examining a Clinical Research Enterprise coordinating activity in which payers, purchasers, patients, investigators, and government agencies work together to examine ways of using for research a national pool of money that superseded, but received contributions from, all the members of the coordinating activity. Would purchasers be interested in participating in this coordinating activity by putting 1% of total health care dollars into a pool that they could direct and use to determine the types of outcomes and ask the kinds of questions that are not currently being addressed?

Money is chemotactic and people will move toward it. We have been considering the concept of not just payers and providers, but also each of the governmental agencies that funds this effort, and potentially the Pharmaceutical Research and Manufacturers of America (PhRMA), the biotechnical industry, pulling together in an evenhanded way, with an economic incentive, to create an infrastructure for the Clinical Research Enterprise. Would purchasers find this method a better way of collectively leveraging the enterprise than what is done now?

Speaker Response to the Enterprise Coordinating Activity Proposal

Helen Darling of the Washington Business Group on Health began the discussion by noting that the concept of a national Clinical Research Enterprise coordinating activity is a good one. She commented that purchasers are changing their role, and that they cannot simply be reactive in the current environment. Jon Hautz of William M. Mercer Inc. also applauded the proposal and asked whether a business case can be made and whether the coordinating activity would add value and not just additional expense. Bruce Taylor of Verizon was intrigued by the idea, noting the breakthrough in funding will come if this coordinating activity becomes a national priority and if the funding comes from a national set-aside. Dale Whitney of United Parcel Service noted that the coordinating activity would provide an additional way for participants to work on the quality dialogue that has currently begun. He noted that those in the corporate office who are responsible for cost containment will want to know what the return will be for this particular investment.

Jill Berger of Marriott mentioned the importance of coordinating the research effort. She noted that purchasers are trying many different approaches to determine what provider and member incentives bring about changes in behavior, but that these efforts are not coordinated. Gregg Lehman, Ph.D. of the National Business Coalition on Health stated that is it hard to argue with a multistakeholder approach to problem solving and concurred that it is a laudable idea. He suggested that the National Quality Forum be a key player in this approach and proposed that a number of roundtable members sit on the purchaser council of the forum. The forum already represents a collaborative effort among the various stakeholders in health care. Dale Whitney noted that before wholly embracing the concept, purchasers need to have a clear picture of what the expected outcomes will be. He concluded that the enterprise coordinating activity will move purchasers from being reactive to proactive and will probably allow the goals of the research community to be accomplished more quickly.

THE IMPORTANCE OF PREVENTION RESEARCH

Hugh Tilson, M.D., Dr.P.H.
Senior Advisor to the Dean
School of Public Health, University of North Carolina

An important question for purchasers is, what is the role of the employer in prevention? Keeping a worker healthy is a better investment; therefore, partnering with local and state public health efforts must part of the employer's strategy. Important questions remain unanswered in the public health practice and systems research agenda. One important question is whether prevention and public health systems research is a priority for the employer.

Bruce Taylor

One view from the health plan perspective is that a member may not stay a member for long. An employer might have the same view, especially in the post-September 11 environment in which downsizing, early retirement, and a variety of other programs are being considered. Both health plans and employers may question what their investment should be in the members' or employees' long-term interest.

There are responsible employers who see the link between prevention and benefit. For example, Verizon has a fairly mature workforce composed of workers who are likely to remain with Verizon throughout their working career and into retirement. The company is interested in how to engage them proactively. That engagement is difficult. Verizon has conducted a few programs—admittedly pilot projects that are not broad-based. One is a healthy babies program and the other involves freedom from back pain. These programs attempt to engage employees or dependents in improving compliance with treatment standards. Verizon provides the coverage absolutely free if individuals follow the prescribed protocols. Initial results show that this approach helps individuals become engaged in their health care.

> There are responsible employers who see the link between prevention and benefit.
>
> —Bruce Taylor

Helen Darling

Most employers believe that prevention can play an important role if it is packaged in appropriate words and not overdone. Talking about preventing disease to improve quality of life and productivity is likely to "hit home." Softening the language can increase employer involvement. The Washington Business Group on Health has a number of projects in partnership with the Centers for Disease Control, in which they are trying to translate prevention information into meaningful messages for their members.

One area in which prevention and public health could become extremely important is the epidemic of obesity in this country. Obesity is a very large problem for employers and results in many negative health consequences. Not nearly enough information is available regarding health risk, the impact of obesity on disease, or effective interventions. Struggling with excess weight is admittedly a difficult problem for many people. In this nation, food is readily available everywhere. Every airport is full of all sorts of rich and fattening foods, and restaurants customarily serve large to enormous portions. This situation poses a public health crisis and ultimately burdens the entire nation.

Jon Hautz, C.E.B.S.

Sometimes the issue of prevention is not brought to the forefront because the focus is on actual health care expenses and not on the potential savings from preventive health behaviors. Choosing to be healthy is a life change, a decision to live differently. Unless the environment changes, the individual is not likely to change. The issue goes beyond what a health plan can provide. Plans can send out all the fliers they want, but if they cannot change the environment

> The issue goes beyond what a health plan can provide. Plans can send out all the fliers they want, but if they cannot change the environment in which the individual makes lifestyle decisions, they will not be able to reinforce the switch to healthier behaviors.
>
> —Jon Hautz

in which the individual makes lifestyle decisions, they will not be able to reinforce the switch to healthier behaviors.

George Isham, M.D.
Medical Director and Chief Health Officer
HealthPartners

Prevention is a cost issue for employers as well. For example, employees at the extreme of the body mass index chart, at 35 or 40, may incur substantial costs associated with bypass operations needed to treat heart conditions related to diabetes. The expenditure for operations such as these is so large that it overwhelms all existing preventive budgets.

Many links that are known to be associated with overweight have no good studies, however, and funding is not forthcoming. There is an extreme dearth of funding for health promotion and disease prevention. Employers are encouraged to use whatever language is required to promote interest in this issue, and they are encouraged to pursue the appropriate funding of not only the obesity issue but also the activity issue and the tobacco issue.

CONSUMER INVOLVEMENT

Myrl Weinberg, C.A.E.
President
National Health Council

In this meeting and in many others, there is much discussion of the increasing role of the patient or consumer in influencing the health care system and the delivery system, particularly with respect to what health care is provided. In nearly every case, however, when meeting participants discuss convening groups of stakeholders to identify problems, examine the challenges, set priorities, and come up with solutions, they mention every stakeholder except the consumer or patient. Discussion often centers on shifting costs to the consumer or patient, or potentially shifting decision-making responsibility to them, but very little is said about working together with them on these issues. When an employer has the primary responsibility for the health care decisions for its employees, these employees should be included the design of the plan.

Helen Darling

Thirty years of health policy in this country has shown that it is difficult to identify consumers or a consumer. Good literature exists to guide proper selection when employees wish to involve consumers in decision making. Large- and medium-sized employers do much surveying of their employees. Most employers consider themselves in frequent contact with their employees, retirees, and dependents. E-mail and the Internet have made possible a constant feedback loop in most corporations. Involving consumers in the changes that have been discussed is possible, but it is difficult.

Increases in health care costs for the coming year have been estimated at close to 14%. This estimate does not take into account either the impact of the events of September 11 or the potential effect of passage of the health care legislation currently before Congress. The actual dollars that consumers will have to pay for health care next year, on a monthly basis and a cost-sharing basis, will be two to four times more than a year or two ago. Consumers will take action because they will be spending much more of their money on health care than before.

Dale Whitney

The switch to a consumer-driven health care system will occur over a number of years. For UPS employees, the switch has been taking place over the last few years and will continue. The company's role is to provide employees with information and the tools that they need to work with their physicians, and within their health care plans, to make effective decisions. Some employees are ready to do that today; some are challenging their physicians regarding their treatment plans. Others will not do that five years from now. They will still want the physician to dictate their treatment plan.

> The switch to a consumer-driven health care system will occur over a number of years.
>
> —Dale Whitney

Many employers survey their employees on a regular basis regarding benefits. UPS conducts annual surveys and multiple focus groups. Some questions discussed are, how do you use the health care system, how can we best help you to use the health care system, and what do we need to change in the way we provide benefits?

PUBLICATION OF A RESEARCH PRIORITIES PROPOSAL

Richard Rettig of RAND started a discussion regarding publication of a clinical research priorities proposal by noting that an asset for purchasers and payers is an immense amount of claims data, which provide a running account of the annual burden of disease in this country. He asked if it might be possible for purchasers and payers to compile an annual statement of 5 to 10 high priority clinical research projects that purchasers would like to see conducted in the coming year. He suggested the statement be published in the *Journal of the American Medical Association* or the *New England Journal of Medicine*. Medical researchers typically set the priorities for clinical research. He suggested that purchasers and payers consider entering the discussion of priority setting for clinical research, thus strengthening the demand for research that pertains to improved clinical practice.

Bruce Taylor responded that employers do have "piles" of data but they do not have the resources or clinical knowledge to convert the data into information, knowledge and appropriate actions. Verizon has looked for researchers with whom to partner and has located some who are willing to help identify key questions. However, few researchers take up the offer. Many employers, including Verizon, would welcome this type of partnership, because it leverages the information that is already available.

Jon Hautz mentioned that sometimes the data that purchasers hope to find is buried in a variety of systems that do not "talk" to each other, and sometimes the quality of the data is poor. Purchasers sometimes discover that the information technology infrastructure is not as robust as expected.

Helen Darling stated that an examination of health care utilization reinforces much that has been brought out in the workshop. Many people are not getting the care that they should. No more research is needed to verify that issue. From the age of the workforce and the distribution, it is possible to determine the most prevalent diseases and the most commonly prescribed drugs. The diseases in older workers are heart disease, cancer, diabetes, gastrointestinal disorders, and depression, not necessarily in that order. In a younger population, the diseases are depression, allergies, asthma, as well as accidents many emergency department visits. Obesity will be at the top of the list for new research in the future.

SUMMARY

The goal of the session on the role of purchasers in the Clinical Research Enterprise was to shed light on how the Clinical Research Enterprise can better serve purchasers as they strive to provide high-quality, affordable health care benefits to employees, retirees, and dependents. Representatives from corporations (General Motors Corporation, United Parcel Service, Marriott International, and William M. Mercer, Inc.) and from business organizations (the National Business Coalition on Health and the Washington Business Group on Health) presented their views on what purchasers need from the Clinical Research Enterprise, how the enterprise has met purchasers' needs, and what purchasers are willing to contribute to the enterprise (see box).

The representatives of the purchaser organizations also examined the problems of translating basic research findings into clinical guidelines, translating clinical recommendations into best evidence-based practice, and providing consumers with accurate information to guide their health and health care choices. They responded to a proposal presented by William Crowley of Harvard University for a National Clinical Research Enterprise Coordinating Activity, in which purchasers, payers, investigators, consumers, and government agencies would contribute to a national fund and would collectively direct and use the fund to examine research questions of national significance that are not currently being addressed. They explored the role of purchasers in furthering research in preventive health care and in encouraging members to adopt healthier lifestyles. They discussed the imminent shift to a consumer-driven health care system in the U.S.A. and the implications of that shift for purchasers. Finally, they considered the usefulness of compiling and publishing a list of clinical research projects that purchasers and payers consider top priority.

Highlights of the Session on the Role of Purchasers in the Clinical Research Enterprise

What do purchasers need from the Clinical Research Enterprise?
- Purchasers need research that can inform benefit design decisions as well as research that sheds light on what they can do to better understand clinical variation and to implement programs that address inappropriate variation. They need to know which new technological innovations and treatments have been proven efficacious through high-quality empirical evidence. They need further research to help them put incentive programs into place that support clinical quality and efficiency.
- Studies providing such evidence must be well designed, well executed, and published in peer-reviewed journals. To make budgetary room for new technology and treatments, the Clinical Research Enterprise must apply rigorous standards of evidence to identify and drive out ineffective or less-than-effective treatments or technology. The Clinical Research Enterprise needs to address the blocks in translating basic research findings into clinically meaningful recommendations and in translating those recommendations into action.
- Purchasers need to understand why agreed-upon clinical practices are not always performed. They need to know why there is wide variation in clinical practice and what solutions can be developed collaboratively to reduce this variation.
- Purchasers are concerned about rising pharmaceutical costs and need unbiased comparisons of new versus existing therapeutic agents.
- The Clinical Research Enterprise needs to encourage physicians and hospitals to incorporate current technology into their practices.
- The Clinical Research Enterprise needs to provide a mechanism for fast-track review for priority research issues.
- The Clinical Research Enterprise must provide better protection against genetic discrimination in insurance coverage and in the workplace.

What are purchasers willing to contribute to the Clinical Research Enterprise?
- Purchasers help disseminate information to consumers on best clinical practices, and they reward hospitals, physicians, and others who are willing to meet best-practice standards.
- Purchasers are willing to pay for quality in health care, but they need to know what they will receive for their investment.
- Some purchasers participate in partnerships with researchers, physicians, and pharmaceutical manufacturers; such efforts can provide guidance on realignment of incentives for providers and employees.
- In the shift to a consumer-driven health care system, purchasers can play a role in preventive health by educating their members and encouraging healthy lifestyle behaviors.
- Purchasers may be interested in contributing to a national fund used to examine research questions of national significance, but they need to know what the return would be for the investment.

2

The Role of Payers in the Clinical Research Enterprise

INTRODUCTION
Sean Tunis, M.D., M.Sc.
Workshop Co-Chair
Director, Coverage and Analysis Group
Office of Clinical Standards and Quality
Centers of Medicare and Medicaid Services
and
Allan Korn, M.D.
Workshop Co-Chair
Senior Vice President and Chief Medical Officer
Blue Cross and Blue Shield Association

Two separate but distinct themes have emerged during the first part of the workshop regarding issues faced by purchasers, and each has different implications for the Clinical Research Enterprise. One theme is the notion of following best practices, following clinical guidelines, and reducing variations in care when the best thing to do is actually known. For example, treating heart attack patients with aspirin, with beta blockers, is the right thing to do, and yet this treatment is not given consistently. The central issue is how to translate that research into practice. This issue in turn has implications for determining what sorts of research studies and interventions the Clinical Research Enterprise ought to be conducting and figuring out what barriers exist to improving quality of care, changing physician behavior, monitoring variations in care, and so forth.

The other theme is how to improve care when the best thing to do is unknown. It is not known, for example, whether new-generation antibiotics lead to similar or better outcomes for patients with chronic obstructive pulmonary disease or emphysema exacerbation than the old inexpensive generic antibiotics. A head-to-head study of any novel antibiotic versus Bactrim or amoxycillin has not been done. The lack of such comparison studies marks a huge failing of the Clinical Research Enterprise. In this part of the workshop, payers will examine how they are affected by each of these issues and will explore their relationship with the Clinical Research Enterprise.

WHAT PAYERS NEED FROM THE CLINICAL RESEARCH ENTERPRISE

Eric Book, M.D.
Chief Medical Officer
Wellmark

Wellmark Blue Cross Blue Shield is a mutual insurer, predominantly in Iowa and South Dakota. The company insures roughly half of the population in Iowa and about a third of the population in South Dakota. As a payer, Wellmark is "caught between a rock and a hard place" in these times of double-digit inflation in medical costs. Purchasers ask payers what they are going to do about this problem. Payers do have some control over the unit cost but not much control over volume.

> The company does not want to be pushed into providing coverage, either by public opinion or by the courts, when a treatment has not been proven, has not demonstrated a cost-effective outcome, or has had deleterious effects on patients.
>
> —Eric Book

Payers have two main questions concerning new products that to come to market: Why are we not paying less? Why are we not being given consideration with regard to the investment that we have already made in the development of the products and procedures being brought to market? These inquiries lead to the next question: What do payers expect to get from the enterprise? The short answer is structure and discipline or, said another way, a demonstration that the dollars are being spent wisely. Wellmark is receiving a greater number of requests from members to fund experimental or new procedures or interventions. These requests often concern terminal illnesses or those for which conventional care has not worked. The company does not want to be pushed into providing coverage, either by public opinion or by the courts, when a treatment has not been proven, has not demonstrated a cost-effective outcome, or has had deleterious effects on patients. An example is autologous bone marrow transplant for breast cancer.

What payers want from the Clinical Research Enterprise is evidence of disciplined and robust management. They would like some individual or some entity to be accountable for the "big picture." They need assurance that the focus of research is appropriately prioritized and managed for cost-effective outcomes.

George Isham, M.D.
Medical Director and Chief Health Officer
HealthPartners

Payers appreciate the current product of the Clinical Research Enterprise in terms of the new treatments and new procedures that help our members and patients obtain better health care and attain better health. What payers need are products and methods that improve the care of patients when they are sick, improve the overall health of individuals when they are well, and help prevent disease. They need to know from the enterprise what works and what does not work, with emphasis on what does not.

Organizational research, such as that in the business schools, needs to be incorporated into the Clinical Research Enterprise. Two recent reports by the Institute of Medicine's Committee on Quality Health Care in America, *To Err is Human: Building a Safer Health System* (2000) and *Crossing the Quality Chasm: A New Health System for the 21st Century* (2001), eloquently call for a system of care. Health care itself is a system of individual solo entrepreneurs and practitioners who need help in making that transformation. Payers need more research on how to be a system of care, and the Clinical Research Enterprise can make the appropriate linkages. Payers are also concerned with how to transform the culture of existing medical practice from a profession-centered, largely individual activity to something resembling a team sport that focuses on patient needs.

> Payers need to know from the enterprise what works and what does not work, with emphasis on what does not.
>
> —George Isham

The culture of the individual medical professional has brought much that is positive to the health of this country over the last century, but the country is now facing the limits of some of the professional precepts. More research is needed on how the professional culture interacts with technology and how medicine can be transformed into a different culture. More needs to be known about population-based community methods of improving individual and community health. Knowledge of community preventive health is lacking. Few research funds are channeled to health promotion and disease prevention relative to the funds spent for treatment. If money is chemotactic, it is drawing most of the attention to the sick end of the spectrum. Although effective treatments are needed and appreciated, some money and attention must be drawn to the other end of the spectrum.

The research community needs ob-

> Payers are also concerned with how to transform the culture of existing medical practice from a profession-centered, largely individual activity to something resembling a team sport that focuses on patient needs.
>
> —George Isham

jective measures for evaluating which research projects are of high quality and which are not. The information needs to be much more transparent than it is today, and it should be available to the public as well as to payers and purchasers. We need to know which trials are safe and which are not, and which research is subject to conflict of interest. The research community also needs a broader perspective on the ethics involved in funding research than is customarily given to researchers. One issue of importance to researchers is the ethics of competing for money at any price relative to other social goods such as affordable health care and equity of distribution of health across the population. These are the ethical issues with which payers wrestle in trying to provide affordable, cost-effective care; yet they seem to be "off the table," in large part, for many individual researchers.

In Minnesota, Wellmark has seven methods of providing preventive care to children and adolescents. These methods are promoted by the federal government through the Early and Periodic Screening, Diagnosis, and Treatment Program; through the state Medicaid program's local program; through the American Academy of Pediatrics, which has one view; through the American Academy of Family Practice, which has another; through the consortium of health practitioners that have come together in the Institute of Clinical Systems Improvement, which has yet another; and through other organizations. It is ironic that although the federal government has done well in funding the research on preventive services for children and adolescents through its task force on clinical preventive services, sponsored by the Agency for HealthCare Research and Quality, much of the information does not find its way into the requirements of the programs that provide health care to children in Minnesota.

Whenever possible, federal and state governments should work towards unified requirements. There ought to be some research into how to create better governmental mechanisms for balancing science with other competing interests. Other important research areas are differential characteristics of populations of poor, underserved children; the frequency of their needs and diseases; and the influence of standards of care relative to the influence in well-off and well-insured populations.

Reed Tuckson, M.D.
Chief Medical Officer
United Healthgroup

United Healthgroup is among the largest of the national health care insurers. One of its major business units is a company called Ingenix, which, among other things, conducts clinical research. A view from the payer perspective is that currently the Clinical Research Enterprise is not focused enough. Greater leadership is needed to help coordinate and focus research activity in a climate of limited resources. The Clinical Research Roundtable is a critical forum for providing this leadership. The members of the roundtable should be very vocal in putting forward a relevant and focused point of view. The time is right. The bioterrorism issues before us demonstrate the need to integrate epidemiology and disease surveillance and connect the data with identification of people at risk. In turn, those data must be connected with the recognition of appropriate therapy; long-term compliance; efficient use of resources; coordination across disciplines; and coordination among employers, health plans, and government. The moment has arrived to bring all of these components together.

> Greater leadership is needed to help coordinate and focus research activity in a climate of limited resources.
>
> —Reed Tuckson

Payers need researchers to decide which studies they should devote their resources to exploring, and they need leadership in that regard. How will they know whether the resulting improvements are worth the effort? What is the process by which they make those choices and those decisions? They do not have a vehicle in place that allows that analysis. The process of prioritizing and funding research projects today is not systematic. Too often research is guided, for example, by what a junior faculty member at "Obscure University Number Three" wants to examine. In addition, payers need to know how new interventions or therapies compare with those that are already available.

Government needs to do a much better job of leadership and of standardizing protocols across different agencies—for example, protocols for mammography or breast self-examination for women at various ages. The organization of clinical research needs to be enhanced. A specific need is to increase the speed with which products are delivered to the market. The current infrastructure does not deliver its products quickly, and it is inefficient from a cost standpoint. The cost structure is caught up in all kinds of competing needs, with much waste. What is needed is better integration of the discovery, development, and commercialization of new interventions. This integration should provide feedback that leads to better and more precise use of newly introduced technologies.

> The process of prioritizing and funding research projects today is not systematic. Too often research is guided, for example, by what a junior faculty member at "Obscure University Number Three" wants to examine.
>
> —Reed Tuckson

The integration needs to include studies of actual use of these technologies by physicians and patients, and that feature has to be built into the model. Often it seems that new products are introduced, and then we wait to see what happens later. Payers want these features to be built in as a continuum. The reality of chronic disease must be recognized, and the coordination of multidisciplinary teams that are centered on the needs of the patient must be encouraged. The

> The organization of clinical research needs to be enhanced. A specific need is to increase the speed with which products are delivered to the market.
>
> —Reed Tuckson

research infrastructure needs to be modeled on that new reality. The incorporation of clinical research into practice is still a major challenge.

Payers need much better sources and integration of information that include performance data. Much more emphasis must be placed on the life-long learning of clinicians, so that they can incorporate these data and are able to use them. Much more attention must be given to the rewards for using the data, whether the rewards come through Continuing Medical Education, board certification, or board recertification, or whether the reward is becoming a "five-star doctor."

Similarly, consumers must have information that informs them about what they should be asking for in their health care coverage. They need to know how to make decisions about choice, not only with regard to elements in their plan, but also with respect to choice of hospitals and physicians on the basis of some sense of evidence of performance. The methodology currently available for determining quality at the level of the individual physician has is inadequate. Employers are beginning to ask the health plans to make individual physician ratings available on the employers' Internet sites. Employers need leadership from the profession, through health services research and other valid measures, to determine how people can be informed legitimately about quality and be fair to physicians.

Robert McDonough, M.D.
Medical Director for Quality Management
Aetna U.S. Healthcare

Aetna U.S. Healthcare is a large national private health insurer that has about 18 million members. In addition to health benefits, Aetna offers dental benefits, vision benefits, life insurance, disability benefits, global health- and other health-related benefits. Its top clinical research priorities are to identify interventions, particularly at the health plan level, that are effective in improving health outcomes and in making more efficient use of health resources (by reducing costs while maintaining or improving health outcomes).

> Few clinical studies compare medical technologies of known effectiveness to one another. . . . New devices are often introduced into the market with little evidence of efficacy.
>
> —Robert McDonough

Health plans can play a role in encouraging dissemination of medical technologies of proven safety and effectiveness. To accomplish this objective, they need studies that evaluate new medical technologies, and studies that new technologies with older established technologies. Few clinical studies compare medical technologies of known effectiveness to one another. In the absence of direct comparative studies, it is difficult, if not impossible, to determine which of several medical interventions are safest and most effective for a particular indication.

Safety and efficacy studies tend to focus on new technologies, and the comparative effectiveness to older established technologies has often been overlooked. Private research funding has focused on clinical studies of new, patentable medical technologies such as new drugs and medical devices. This focus leaves out many developments, such as new surgical procedures and physical therapy maneuvers that do not involve a patentable technology. Private research funding for that kind of research is lacking, yet it is important research.

> Payers need health services research that examines methods of organizing the health delivery, both to increase the efficiency and to improve the organization of care.
>
> —Robert McDonough

Food and Drug Administration requirements for devices are much weaker than those for drugs. New devices are often introduced into the market with little evidence of efficacy. They often are promoted heavily, and pressure for coverage is enormous. Health plans try to hold the line and insist on evidence of effectiveness. Frequently that evidence is not forthcoming, and at some point comes the realization that the intervention is not effective at all.

Evidence-based clinical practice guidelines and consensus statements have often been used by health plans in making coverage decisions. Cost-effectiveness analyses have only been applied to primary clinical preventive services. Payers have not reached the point where they perform cost-effectiveness analyses to decide to cover new technologies that are proven to offer a clinically significant benefit. Cost is only taken into account in coverage decisions where there are two or more equally effective medical interventions for a given indication. Payers need health services research that examines methods of organizing the health delivery, both to increase the efficiency and to improve the organization of care.

Chuck Cutler, M.D.
Chief Medical Officer
American Association of Health Plans

Research on the effectiveness of prevention is an example of the kind of research that is helpful to health plans. A fair amount about the cost-effectiveness of preventive care services is known. Virtually all health plans have put a substantial amount of energy into improving preventive care services, even though many of these services do not provide cost savings to the health plan.

Payers should look more broadly at the research topics and examine not only whether something works but what its benefits are—benefits not just in terms of medical care cost savings but also to society.

A question that has been raised is whether the funding of clinical research is sufficient. While it is difficult to answer that question, there is always more valuable research to be done and other equally worthy activities to fund. One clear problem that emerges is the prioritization of clinical research. The goal of the Clinical Research Enterprise should be to improve the health of the American people. At the present time, it appears that politics and traditional drive some of the research endeavors, and the political process also drives some of the funding. It is not clear how the rest of the funding priorities are decided. Bringing a more transparent, rational decision-making process to the funding process would be an improvement. The Institute of Medicine report *Crossing the Quality Chasm* suggests a prioritization for research activities that is focused on disease burden, and the research activity should be structured in the manner that would be most likely to decrease the disease burden.

In order to decide what services to cover and recommend, health plans need information about what works and what does not. Health plans also provide an infrastructure to support improvements in care that is otherwise lacking in the American health care system. They have a large interest in clinical trials. To some degree, they also provide an infrastructure to support improvements in care that is otherwise lacking in the American health care system. So they need to know where to invest their energies to gain the greatest improvements in outcomes for the populations they serve and which interventions will produce the best results.

> Currently under-funded [areas of clinical research are] operational research, information technology research, research on how to get people to change their behaviors in a clinical setting, and how to provide the appropriate information systems and other supports in a clinical setting.
>
> —Chuck Cutler

Clinical research endeavors have significant safety problems. Payers have been concerned that insufficient safety controls are in place in the Clinical Research Enterprise and that many patients participating in clinical research are subject to avoidable risks. The clinical research enterprise needs to assure adequate oversight of clinical trials to protect patient safety. About 15 years is needed to put innovations that are proven to be effective into practice. Health plans need a better understanding of how to move these innovations into practice and how to be part of the Clinical Research Enterprise. That effort to translate research and innovation into practice would include areas that are currently under-funded, e.g., operational research, information technology research, research on how to get people to change their behaviors in a clinical setting, and how to provide the appropriate information systems and other supports in a clinical setting.

The research community could learn much by examining how industries have improved their operations. The health care community seems to be focused parochially on clinical research and has continued to follow a traditional research agenda. We need to know more about behavioral factors in care. We need to understand what the behavioral barriers are. We can address access barriers where they exist, but there are other barriers that we do not understand. Health literacy barriers are problematic, and additional research in this area is needed.

Appropriate incentives are needed to encourage providers and researchers to investigate how to translate research into practice. The main way in which information is currently disseminated is through traditional venues, e.g., professional journal publication. Research is needed on how to improve the delivery of innovations that we know are effective, and information about these innovations needs to be disseminated through new, more effective means. To protect patients, we also need more rigorous standards for innovations that do not require FDA approval, such as surgical procedures. Devices, even with FDA approval, are loosely evaluated and may not be safe or effective.

Finally, an important issue is patient-centeredness. More patients will be making decisions about what kind of care they receive. They already are making those decisions. Right now, physicians see patients who bring in stacks of printouts from the Internet about new therapies and factors that they should consider.

Payers need measures and information that patients can use to evaluate their care. Similarly, few measures exist for physicians and others to use for evaluating their performance. Most physicians in practice probably measure very little in the population they serve, other than through the data that they receive from health plans or perhaps from hospitals. The situation needs to change, and payers need guidance from the Clinical Research Enterprise as to what measures are important, what will bring the greatest improvement in the health of the American people, and what support to provide to physicians to promote these changes. We depend on the Clinical Research Enterprise to develop, test, and evaluate new interventions to determine if they are safe and effective as well as how they compare to existing interventions. These interventions should include the widest range of services including not only new technologies, but educational, counseling, and other services as well.

WHAT PAYERS ARE WILLING TO CONTRIBUTE TO THE CLINICAL RESEARCH ENTERPRISE

Robert McDonough, M.D.

Health plans can contribute to the Clinical Research Enterprise by directly funding research. An example of an effective partnership that has produced worthwhile results is Aetna's Academic Medicine and Managed Care Forum, which was founded by Aetna to foster a closer working relationship between academic medicine and managed care. Participants now include 53 of the nation's top medical institutions, medical societies, major employers, federal agencies, private foundations, pharmaceutical companies, and medical professional organizations. The forum provides an arena where participants can collaboratively influence the delivery of high-quality medical care through the forum's three principal components: working groups, research funding, and semiannual meetings. The forum includes a Quality Care Research Fund, initiated in 1997 with a $15 million commitment from Aetna. Between 1997 and 2000, over $26 million was awarded for research. The types of studies that have been funded by the forum are described on its website, www.academicforum.org.

Health plans help put clinical research findings into practice through disease management efforts, provider education initiatives, and other programs. Health plans also disseminate clinical research findings and evidence-based guidelines to physicians. Aetna distributes tens of thousands of continuing medical education monographs to its physicians, and it provides financial incentives to physicians to participate in continuing medical education. It distributes clinical practice guidelines that are based on evidence-based guidelines of medical professional organizations, and preventative structure guidelines that are based on the work of the U.S. Preventive Services Task Force. Aetna also has its InteliHealth professional website, which provides constant flow of information that is available to all physicians, not just its participating physicians.

> Health plans help put clinical research findings into practice through disease management efforts, provider education initiatives, and other programs.
>
> —Robert McDonough

Aetna disseminates health information to its members through its member health education program, InteliHealth website, and its Informed Health nurse help line. These services help empower consumers to obtain the information that they need for making health care decisions.

Aetna develops evidence-based clinical coverage policies and uses the results of evidence-based research to make coverage decisions objectively. The tools that health plans use to help provide incentives for promoting evidence-based medicine are preauthorization, pre-certification, the pharmacy formulary, concurrent review, and retrospective review. Also, quality improvement programs involve measurement of adherence to clinical guidelines, feedback on the results, and provision of incentives to physicians. Clinical programs are used to identify and assure provision of appropriate evidence-based care to members with special health care needs. These are disease management programs that deal with specific diseases, case management programs that focus on people with critical illnesses, and maternity management programs.

Health plans can also help implement the results of clinical research into clinical practice by encouraging enrollment of patients in FDA-approved clinical trials. Aetna and many other health plans cover promising experimental treatments for patients with life-threatening illness who are being treated as part of a protocol in an FDA-approved clinical trial. Health plans may cover some costs of clinical trials besides those for life-threatening illnesses. Many health plans cover routine care costs for patients who are enrolled in clinical trials. Medicare and many health plans cover Category B investigational devices, which involve incremental modifications to established devices.

Finally, health plans have an opportunity to create networks of care that can steer patients to centers that use evidence-based protocols and attain superior clinical outcomes. Aetna's National Medical Excellence Program reviews institutions' evidence-based protocols and clinical outcomes data to select those preferred centers for organ transplantation and for management of complex cases.

Health plans are important consumers of research on clinical effectiveness, comparative effectiveness, cost effectiveness, and the effectiveness of the organization and delivery of health services. Health plans can support the Clinical Research Enterprise by funding clinical research directly and indirectly by using the tools available to them to promote the translation of clinical research results into clinical practice.

> Health plans can also help implement the results of clinical research in clinical practice by encouraging enrollment of patients in FDA-approved clinical trials.
>
> —Robert McDonough

There are arguments for both private (e.g., health plan) and public funding for research on interventions at the health plan level for improving efficiency and health outcomes. Health plans have an obligation to fund this research. But public funding should also be provided because the general public benefits from research on the organization and delivery of health care, and the results of this research may improve the efficiency of health care delivery and improve health care outcomes.

> Health plans have an opportunity to create networks of care that can steer patients to centers that use evidence-based protocols and attain superior clinical outcomes.
>
> —Robert McDonough

Eric Book, M.D.

Most Blue Cross Blue Shield plans provide benefit coverage for clinical trials. In October 1998, the Blue Cross and Blue Shield Association board passed a recommendation that member health plans pay up to the member's benefit level for participation in a clinical trial, and 88% of Blue Cross Blue Shield members now receive this benefit. Another 7% to 8% receive coverage for clinical trial participation on request or on appeal.

Once a new technology comes to market, has been proven, and becomes accepted, it tends to be priced much higher than the technologies that it replaces. The reason given is that the additional revenue funds research and development of these drugs and continuing research. Finally, a large amount of tax revenue is used for research.

George Isham, M.D.

Healthpartners, like many other payers, is directly involved in clinical research. Its research priorities are as follows:

- Heart disease, diabetes, and depression
- Obesity and its prevention
- Promotion of physical activity in the population
- Elimination of smoking
- Development of a system of prevention, health promotion, and clinical care
- Development of community and population approaches to improving the members' health
- Development of methods for improving patient safety and avoidance of errors in care
- Applying methods of care known to be effective and eliminating unsafe and ineffective care

RESEARCH PRIORITIES AND PRIORITY SETTING FOR PAYERS

Myron Genel of Yale University School of Medicine began the discussion of research priorities by pointing out that many of the points made about translational blocks earlier in the workshop concerned the second translational block, putting clinical research into practice, rather than the first block, translating basic research into clinical research. He noted that in the first area, the traditional investigator-initiated research project has thrived in this country because it has created the ferment that allows great ideas to percolate. In contrast, it appears that this approach does not work in the second area. Other speakers have suggested that a more industrial model is needed at the second bottleneck to circumvent the disincentives that exist. At the first level, one cannot predict what research will be important, and too great a focus at that level might shut off the out-of-the-way idea that later proves to be fruitful. A more focused effort at the more pragmatic second-level bottleneck may be appropriate, however.

Reed Tuckson of United Healthgroup mentioned that it is possible to focus the Clinical Research Enterprise and set priorities without inhibiting investigator-initiated research. From a national perspective, efforts should be focused on the largest disease burden. He suggested that there is a need to track research questions and their answers in an integrated way that puts all the pieces together from inception, rather than to look at the pieces individually and hope that somewhere along the line they will fall into a nice mosaic.

Lewis Sandy of the Robert Wood Johnson Foundation stated that purchasers and payers understand the term "research" differently than investigators do. Purchasers and payers usually use the term to mean the application of analytic methods to solve business problems, whereas investigators use it to mean asking and answering questions or testing hypotheses. Sometimes those two meanings intersect, but sometimes they do not.

> Purchasers and payers understand the term "research" differently than investigators do. Purchasers and payers usually use the term to mean the application of analytic methods to solve business problems, whereas investigators use it to mean asking and answering questions or testing hypotheses. Sometimes those two meanings intersect, but sometimes they do not.
>
> —Lewis Sandy

Lewis Sandy noted a paradox in the discussion: purchasers and payers have expressed a need for more information about what works and why, as well as a need for more outcome research, and have noted that the process of research is slow and laborious and does not fit their timeframes for decision making. Yet the laboratory for asking and answering such questions is the world of practice, change, and purchaser behavior, as well as the world of delivery systems, which purchasers and payers collectively represent. The RWJ Foundation funds, as does AHRQ and others, the work of many investigators who want to answer the kinds of questions purchasers and payers raise; yet investigators find that task challenging because the world is changing in a chaotic way that does not allow asking and answering questions or testing hypotheses. Sandy asked purchasers and payers: when you make changes in your system, would you consider using random assignment or quasi-experimental designs that would allow health services and outcome researchers to ask and answer questions and provide you with the answers that you say you would like?

Chuck Cutler of the American Association of Health Plans mentioned that health plans do hypothesis testing of research ideas regularly, sometimes through formal investigation as in collaborative research with universities, and other times from a more formal practical business case analysis. Health plans are interested in questions such as the following: What are the causes of disease? What are the potential interventions? Are they successful or not?

> Health plans are interested in more than just a business research model.
>
> —Chuck Cutler

Health plans are interested in more than just a business research model, however. A number of health plans are directly involved in research that is funded by NIH, AHRQ, the Veterans Administration (VA), and other agencies. In fact, more and more health plans are participating in research.

A payer's main purpose, as suggested by George Isham of HealthPartners, is to provide affordable health care to as many people as possible and, as a delivery organization, to provide what is known to be good health care as efficiently and effectively as possible with the highest satisfaction. The main purpose is not necessarily the discovery of new knowledge. Dr. Isham also noted that payers have tremendous opportunities for working together with researchers who are disciplined and trained in methodology, analysis, and study design and who are trying to determine how to deliver the care that is known to be efficacious. New methodologies are needed to answer these questions because the randomized clinical trial cannot always be used, particularly if the number of subjects is small.

Reed Tuckson commented that the questions payers need to ask must represent the interests of many stakeholders and as part of the ultimate public good. Employers should not be expected to jeopardize their financial stability by paying for health care that is not effective. Instead they need to have their questions answered. Bright clinical researchers with expertise in addressing the relevant questions must take the lead in finding answers to these questions. Unless and until they do, measures may be imposed from outside the profession. That is not the way it should happen. There need not be a dichotomy; instead there can be a fluid integration between different interests. For example, United Healthcare sponsors a center for health care policy and research; while completely independent, the researchers live shoulder-to-shoulder with the business people who are trying to answer some of these questions. We know that relevant and practical research can occur in such settings.

> Employers should not be expected to jeopardize their financial stability by paying for health care that is not effective.
>
> —Reed Tuckson

Al Reece, Vice Chancellor and Dean of the University of Arkansas College of Medicine, asked whether payers' interests are so focused that the health benefits need to be short-term. Suppose that the benefits could indeed be long-term, he speculated. For example, some estimates by medical economists have suggested that the savings from osteoporosis prevention could exceed $300 million annually. Although the savings would not show up in the balance book for several years, it would be indeed be substantial.

Chuck Cutler responded that payers need to know whether interventions are safe and effective, where they fit in the hierarchy of other interventions for the same disease, and what the cost implications are. The cost benefits of preventive care services must also be understood. Only a few preventive interventions offer cost savings. All of these have benefit, but the benefits come at some additional cost. Health plans have invested in increasing the use of many of these preventive interventions. Payers also need to understand the costs and benefits associated with disease management programs that help physicians do more than they can individually to provide preventive care and continuing care services for chronic diseases.

George Isham noted that accompanying the decrease of uncompensated care is the increasing use of cost accounting mechanisms to justify the implementation of programs. In his view, going the accounting route totally is not an adequate way to decide which programs should be deployed and which should not. He called for consideration to be given to what social and other mechanisms can be instituted to benefit society as a whole in the long run, stating that a health care organization that invests in the health of its community will benefit in some fashion from its own efforts and those of its competitors.

In the view of Eric Book of Wellmark, it is less important to payers that the outcomes are short-term or long-term and more important that they are tangible. If they are tangible, payers will support them and will do so with the full knowledge their members today may not be their members five years from now.

TRANSLATIONAL BLOCKS

Ken Getz began the discussion of translational blocks in research by asking for examples of instances in which translation of a medical intervention from research into practice actually went smoothly. Panelists were unable to offer any concrete examples.

Chuck Cutler mentioned the use of beta blockers after myocardial infarction as a good example. Health plans and hospitals in some cases have installed systems to detect cases and examine prescription records. Persons not on beta blockers are identified for their physicians so they prescribe them appropriately. Advances in anesthesiology provide an example of identifying major threats to safety and designing industrial solutions. For instance, to eliminate errors, equipment for delivering anesthetic agents has different inputs for oxygen and the anesthetic agent. Other areas in which progress has been made are examinations for retinopathy, foot examinations, and hemoglobin A1c testing in people with diabetes. These efforts are most successful when they are value-added to physicians and when they are systematic. Information on these advances needs to be disseminated to individual physicians.

> [Translational] efforts are most successful when they are value-added to physicians and when they are systematic.
>
> —*Chuck Cutler*

Reed Tuckson mentioned diabetes care as an example in which all legitimate expert opinions have been heard and organizations have worked together to develop integrated performance measures. The cooperating organizations range from the American Diabetes Association (ADA); to specialty societies for endocrinology, internal medicine, and family practice; all the way to health plans and the Joint Commission on Accreditation of Healthcare Organizations.

Veronica Catanese of New York University School of Medicine gave the example of achieving normal glycosylated hemoglobin and pointed out that, although practice guidelines are well defined, the essential components for accomplishing this goal are not always in place. There are missing links in terms of how we enable the patients to achieve the goal. What is needed is behavior change, technology, counseling, and family support, among other factors. In response, Hugh Tilson of the University of North Carolina School of Public Health suggested that some partnerships outside the health care delivery system, in the public health system, might be useful in bringing about the desired change.

The practical application of these initiatives can be interesting, replied Eric Book. As are many health plans, Wellmark is interested in reducing variation among physician practices. In Iowa Wellmark attempted to emulate the Minnesota model and to see if all major insurers and provider organizations could agree on a single guideline in a disease entity, and diabetes was chosen. They were very successful in agreeing on implementing a statewide guideline. The problem was that physician behavior was not substantially affected. A greater effect was achieved by working with the people with diabetes rather than with the physicians. When we focused directly on those with diabetes we started to see behavioral changes.

Hal Slavkin of the University of Southern California School of Dentistry called for including a broader set of stakeholders if large gains are to be made in improving quality of life, reducing incidence of disease, and decreasing health disparities. He noted that we may miss a critical opportunity to include those who influence prenatal care and K-12 education in this country if we just use terms such as risk assessment, disease prevention, and health promotion.

John Graham of the American Diabetes Association noted that the ADA is moving aggressively in the area of school lunches because it has noted that the food in the schools is deplorable. Not only does school food have low nutritional value, but the opportunity to buy food is entirely too prevalent. The issue of food in schools cuts across all disease entities.

John Graham noted that the second key area is physical education. Once mandatory for all grade levels, and even for college students, it is now much less visible. Programs such as the President's

---

> Although practice guidelines are well defined . . . there are missing links . . . behavior change, technology, counseling, and family support among other factors.
>
> —Veronica Catanese

Council on Physical Fitness need to be reinstated; we are now paying a price for the lack of physical activity among the country's youth, and the cost will continue to rise. The ADA is moving forward to work with the administration and the Department of Agriculture on those two issues.

A discussion of these larger issues poses some risk of running well ahead of the evidence, warned Robert Califf of Duke University School of Medicine. He cited diet as an example of an area in which implementing broad public policies may turn out to be detrimental. For instance, the low-fat diet that has been promoted as beneficial for the heart, has been misinterpreted by the public, leading to a major increase in consumption of carbohydrate, causing obesity and diabetes.

Allan Korn of the Blue Cross Blue Shield Association mentioned that the FDA has a good process for the adoption of new drugs. When pharmaceutical agents are proven to be safe and effective, they are rapidly adopted by health plans and made available. Where the system breaks down is the stampede to allow use of the drug for other conditions than those indicated in order to increase market share rapidly. This process can proceed smoothly, but if focus and discipline are not maintained, it can break down along the way.

George Isham noted that the payer and purchaser community adopts guidelines developed by AHRQ, or policy announcements by Medicare or Medicaid in the states, but that many factors other than evidence and research come into play. Better models are needed for how the government can make linkages between evidence and practice. It is high time that the government stepped forward and took on this issue. As important as private purchasers have been in driving the use of good science and evidence over the last 10 years, the leading purchasers represent only a small sector of the great mass of private purchasers, more and more of whom are unaware of these issues and ineffective in driving change in local markets.

David Rimoin of the Cedar-Sinai Medical Center, cautioned against assuming that once something is unambiguously demonstrated to be effective, it will be adopted. He described working in a system with 200 full-time physicians and 2,000 attending staff physicians who are fiercely independent "lonesome cowboys." In this climate, information technology may be a key to the standardization of effective practices. Once a guideline received approval, it could become the standard and "roll out" through the electronic medical record and patient billing systems. If a physician did not agree with the standard, the physician would have to make an effort to document his or her reasoning. This system might initially be limited to hospitals because most outpatient facilities and physicians' offices do not have this technology.

Independence among physicians is an important issue, noted Reed Tuckson. If physicians decide that there really is no accountability for quality, and if the physician is not accountable for taking the lead, the question then becomes, who then steps up to the plate? Many employers in the room today, and other leaders around the country, are saying, if no one is going to step up to the plate, we will. They are demanding change. An example is "Leapfrog." What are the boards going to do? What are the specialty societies going to do? Who will step up in the lead from the profession itself? Will it take the employers demanding that we all push this through? It is intellectually dishonest if we do not point out the issues, and if each of us—employers, purchasers, plans, hospitals, individual physicians, medical groups—do not make collective decisions about how we are going to behave and what our accountability is. Ideally, we need a collaborative effort and physicians should lead the way.

Francis Chesley of the Agency for Healthcare Research and Quality noted in response that the government role is not sufficient and that partnerships are essential. The Agency for Healthcare Research and Quality, under its previous name the Agency for Healthcare Policy and Research, had the charge to bring clinical practice guidelines to the fore. As a result of that charge and leadership, that agency almost went out of existence. It is only through partnerships—and the AHRQ has them with the American Medical Association and the American Association with Health Plans—that we have actually been able to accomplish something in terms of bringing evidence-based information to the practitioner level.

Purchasers are already interested in trying to hold physicians accountable at the individual level, stated Patricia Salber of General Motors Corporation. Purchasers are asking physicians to set up information technology systems so that the physician can monitor how he or she is managing patients. The aim is to encourage the physician to not only provide care to the individual patient but also manage the population that is his or her panel.

David Scheinberg of the Memorial Sloan-Kettering Cancer Center described a system that the center established several years ago to try to deal with the issue of standardizing care among a captive group of physicians, all of whom are full-time employees salaried by the corporation. Every patient who entered the institution became a homunculus on a computer system, and all were tracked from the day they walked in to the day they left or died. Every laboratory order, every test, every operation, and every drug administered was tracked, the costs were monitored, and all data were tabulated for every physician and every patient. The system was an effort, at that time, to deal with costs and managed care issues. It turned out that, even in this extraordinarily well controlled, captive audience, every patient was an "N of one" and every patient had a variance. Although plans, drafted over two years, were instituted by the physicians to propose the appropriate and best standard of care for every disease encountered, hundreds of different pathways, mapping every possible pathway, were instituted in this computer, and yet there were still hundreds of variants. That result was in a very small microcosm. The idea of instituting such a system on a community or national level is a laudable goal, but very difficult to achieve, to say the least.

CONSUMER DEMAND

A discussion of the participation of consumers in health care and the resulting impact on payers was begun by Edward Campion of the *New England Journal of Medicine,* who stated that the locus of control seems to be shifting toward the more assertive patients and consumers. In many cases these consumers are basing their decisions largely on health information from the media, which is, at times, directed at them with financial incentives behind it. Consequently, what drugs are dispensed or what operation is performed depends not on consumers' knowledge of results of randomized controlled trials or cost benefit analysis, but on patients' perception of how these treatments will affect them.

Reed Tuckson asserted that the real dilemma is how to address the public education system in America, which helps us train and educate people to understand the complexities underlying modern science. Another important dilemma is how to arm people with the information that they need to be able to give informed consent in the genomic era. The educational system, not the health care system, must deal with those enormous public challenges. It is encouraging that organizations such as the National Health Council are providing the beginnings of fundamental sets of questions and answers to people in all of their organizations, and are emphasizing that consumers are the captains of their own health care teams. These organizations are also recognizing that consumers have the right to make health care choices in the context of their relationships with their physician. The empowering role of the consumer is key, and the means of providing the information is important. Here the Internet plays a major role, although the racial and economic disparities in access to that technology must be recognized. It is clear, though, that we are making progress. Consumers must have access to information that allows them, across a continuum from the most interested to the most passive, to participate intelligently in their health care.

> What drugs are dispensed or what operation is performed depends not on consumers' knowledge of results of randomized controlled trials or cost benefit analysis, but on patients' perception of how these treatments will affect them.
>
> —*Edward Campion*

George Isham noted that the more that consumers are faced with competing information and competing clinical trials in which to participate, the greater will be the need for transparency with respect to the Internal Review Board proceedings, the benefit of the research intervention, and the options available outside of the research trial. Consumerism is often equated to paying the bill, in the sense that there are more co-pays. We find that for more of our insurance and managed care products, purchasers and others are asking us to include more features such as co-insurance and deductibles in the product. This inclination is in direct conflict with the inclusion of all therapeutic elements for diabetes, which was brought up earlier in the workshop. Our thoughts used to be that if it works, it ought to be paid for in a broadly first-dollar coverage insurance product. Apparently many conflicting paradigms exist in the current marketplace as to what an insurance product is or is not, and how consumerism interacts with whether it is right to have consumers pay the bill.

PATIENT PARTICIPATION IN CLINICAL RESEARCH

An issue posed by John Gallin of the National Institutes of Health Clinical Center is how to encourage providers to refer patients to the Clinical Research Enterprise as study participants. Recruitment of patients for participation in clinical studies, whether natural history studies or clinical trials, is increasingly difficult. Patients no longer have the personal relationship with their physician that was prevalent 15 years ago, when nearly all patients knew their physicians, as opposed to only 6 in 10 patients today. Many patients consider their insurance carrier to be their provider, and many worry that they will lose their insurance coverage if they participate in a clinical trial. A common perception among patients is that they would have difficulty obtaining permission to participate in a clinical research activity.

In response, Chuck Cutler noted that barriers to participation in clinical trials are multifactorial and that health plans do not present the greatest barrier. Other barriers are lack of physician awareness of clinical trials, lack of physician willingness to refer patients to clinical trials because the patients will then lose their relationship with the physicians, and patients' unwillingness to be what they perceive as "guinea pigs" in clinical trials. He stated that he did not believe that any health plan would deny someone the opportunity to participate in a study funded by the National Institutes of Health (NIH), depending on the benefit design.

SUMMARY

The goal of the session on the role of purchasers in the Clinical Research Enterprise was to elucidate how the Clinical Research Enterprise can better serve payers as they strive to provide affordable health care coverage to as many people as possible, provide best evidence-based health care efficiently and effectively with the highest satisfaction, and contribute to health care research. Representatives from health plans (Wellmark Blue Cross Blue Shield, Health Partners, United Healthgroup, and Aetna U.S. Healthcare) and a representative from the American Association of Health Plans presented their views on what payers need from the Clinical Research Enterprise, how the enterprise has met payers' needs, and what payers are willing to contribute to the enterprise (see box).

The representatives of the health plan industry also discussed bottlenecks in translation of basic science into clinical practice and the translation of clinical guidelines into care, citing incidences of successful translation of medical interventions from research to practice. They examined the role of health care plans in improving the health care system and advancing the health of the community as a whole. They acknowledged the shift toward greater participation of consumers in their own health care and explored means for enhancing consumer education. Finally, they addressed the concern that health care plans may present barriers to patient participation in clinical trials.

Highlights of the Session on the Role of Payers in the Clinical Research Enterprise

What do payers need from the Clinical Research Enterprise?
- Payers depend on the Clinical Research Enterprise to develop the interventions that will improve the health of the populations they serve and society as a whole. Payers need to understand what works and what does not work in the care of patients, the prevention of disease, and the promotion of health. They need to know how to provide safer care and eliminate errors to keep members free from harm while participating in health care.
- Payers need new knowledge on how to transform health care into a more systematic effort and how to help professionals understand that they are part of this systematic effort. They need to give guidance on how to transform the culture of medical practice from a profession-centered, individual activity into a patient-centered, team activity. They need more insight into population-based community methods of improving individual and community health.
- Payers need to know from the enterprise which research projects are of high quality and which are not, and which research efforts are safe and which are not. They need to know which researchers have conflicts of interest and what those conflicts are. They need full disclosure of information regarding research funding to the public, potential research participants, and other stakeholders.
- Research is needed on the barriers to the delivery of or patient adherence to interventions or behavior change, such as health illiteracy, cultural competencies, insurance issues, financial issues, or transportation issues.

How has the Clinical Research Enterprise met payers' needs?
- The Clinical Research Enterprise provides the knowledge that helps payers understand that what they do for patients is helpful. It provides payers with innovations that improve care, prevent illness, and promote health. The Clinical Research Enterprise holds the potential to question existing practice and help over time to eliminate ineffective and even harmful practices.

What are payers willing to contribute to the Clinical Research Enterprise?
- Payers play a role in encouraging dissemination of medical technologies of proven safety and effectiveness. They can also encourage the implementation of evidence-based guidelines and consensus statements in clinical practice.
- Payers have supported research activities both independently and by forming partnerships with medical institutions, medical societies, employers, federal agencies, private foundations, pharmaceutical companies, and medical professional organizations.
- Payers help put clinical research findings into practice through disease management efforts and provider-education initiatives. They also disseminate health information to their members through health education programs.

3

The Role of Other Stakeholders in the Clinical Research Enterprise

INTRODUCTION

Myrl Weinberg, C.A.E.
President
National Health Council

Now that this workshop has given us a better understanding of the different stakeholders' views, which are legitimate from their perspectives and from the standpoint of their organizations' mission and goals, it is even more imperative that we look for unique solutions that we can work together to apply. We need to think creatively about new ways to address some of the clinical research issues that have been raised.

It is important not to view the stakeholders and the patients as distinct, potentially conflicting, parties. In fact, patients are the ultimate stakeholders of clinical research. A habit ingrained in many of our infrastructures and organizations is to give patients information, and perhaps survey them once in a while, but not to enter into an interactive and respectful dialogue. All decisions about plans, structures, what is paid for and how it is paid for must involve consumers/patients/employees from the very beginning. Simply "keeping them happy" is not appropriate because if they are not involved and educated about the nuances within health care, they may be happy with the wrong things. If we do not involve them up front, they will be involved but perhaps in ways that are not the most effective or appropriate. They may become more and more aggressive and demanding, and the process will not be as productive as a cooperative dialogue would be.

The important role of the consumers should be borne in mind during this part of the workshop as we hear from representatives of voluntary health agencies, the device industry, and the Agency for Healthcare Research and Quality. Panelists from each organization will describe their organization's relationship with the Clinical Research Enterprise, define the organization's contribution to the enterprise, and discuss the organization's needs and concerns related to the research arena.

THE ROLE OF VOLUNTARY HEALTH ASSOCIATIONS IN THE CLINICAL RESEARCH ENTERPRISE

John Stevens, M.D.
Vice President for Extramural Grants, Research Department
American Cancer Society

The American Cancer Society (ACS) has a single purpose, which is to eliminate cancer as a major health problem, and it accomplishes that goal through a variety of programs. The organization is present in 3,400 communities around the country and represents the interests of cancer patients, cancer survivors, and their families. The Clinical Research Enterprise has been critical to the progress that has been made in the cancer arena. Cancer is foremost among the health concerns of the American public, and the disease costs the nation about $180 billion a year.

> The Clinical Research Enterprise has been critical to the progress that has been made in the cancer arena.
>
> —John Stevens

From the perspective of the American Cancer Society, funding for the Clinical Research Enterprise continues to be a high priority. The clinical research enterprise also faces a barrier in dissemination. New therapies and standards of care must be disseminated throughout the health care delivery system in order for them to achieve the goal of improving care.

In addition, many patients have limited access to the fruits of the Clinical Research Enterprise. The new therapies produced by clinical research do not reach enough patients. Barriers to receiving the high quality care that the country can produce include educational barriers, financial barriers (including inadequate insurance coverage for cutting-edge care), and barriers within the health care delivery system that may make accessing high quality care difficult. This is especially true in access among medically underserved communities and populations.

For many cancer patients, all of these barriers may apply. In addition to increased funding for the Clinical Research Enterprise, the American Cancer

Society supports the dissemination of the information learned through clinical research through public health programs, and through increased access to public and private insurance programs, increased access to high quality care at community health centers, adequate coverage to ensure quality care throughout the continuum of cancer care, increased coordination of health care delivery systems to improve dissemination of high quality care, and quality assurance for care.

Other obstacles facing the Clinical Research Enterprise include ensuring the protection and privacy of participants in research involving humans. Improving elements of the drug development process to ensure that new standards of care are available for patients as efficiently as possible is also important.

The ACS has its own research program, which ranges from basic to clinical and applied, including epidemiology, psychosocial research, behavioral research, health policy, and health services research. Advocacy for more research funding is a very important role of the ACS. The ACS has a strong advocacy effort in Washington, D.C., where it joins with other interested organizations under an umbrella called One Voice Against Cancer Together. Representatives from the organizations visit Congress to advocate for increasing the NIH budget and the budget of the National Cancer Institute. The ACS also advocates at the Centers for Disease Control (CDC) for additional funds so that the fruit of this research can be translated into community application. An example would be the breast and cervical detection cancer programs, where the CDC gives block grants to the state health departments.

Consistent with our mission, we have traditionally funded about 80% of what we call basic research in our own program. About 20% is "nonbasic" or applied, which ranges from translational research to investigation at the other end of the spectrum—cancer control, small clinical trials, prevention trials, behavioral trials, and health policy. The ACS is shifting that balance so that it will become 50/50 over the next few years, not by removing funding from basic research, but by adding more resources to the applied side.

The ACS is also very interested in educating the public, the patients, and the professionals as to what is available in state-of-the-art detection, prevention, and treatment. The organization has a 24-hour 800 number in at least two languages for providing information to patients or their families, or to whoever is interested in calling. That number receives about a million calls a year. The ACS also has its own website.

The ACS advocates for high-quality care for all cancer patients, primarily through efforts at the state and federal levels. It also advocates for coverage of the cost of the research component of clinical trials. Further, it advocates for all efforts that will result in decreasing disparities and outcomes among the various patient groups. Not everyone has equal access to health care or equal outcomes in this country. Not only are there differences in how state-of-the-art health care is practiced by different professionals in the U.S.A., but there are also huge regional differences in how health care is administered and practiced. That issue is another area that needs special attention.

John Graham IV
Chief Executive Officer
American Diabetes Association

The mission of the American Diabetes Association is to prevent and cure diabetes and to improve the lives of all people affected by diabetes. Its vision statement is, have we made an everyday difference in the quality of life for people with diabetes? The ADA is unique among voluntary health agencies in that it is actually two organizations in one, which is a benefit. It is the professional society for the 20,000 health professionals who specialize in diabetes—everyone from PhD scientists to practicing clinicians, to nurses and dieticians, to exercise physiologists and pharmacists. It is also the advocate for the more than 16 million Americans who have diabetes. We have banished from our language the term 'diabetic.' We use the term 'people with diabetes' because we believe that people are people and not necessarily diabetics. We do not use the term 'patient,' because it has a victim connotation. Instead we use the term 'people who have a chronic disorder,' with which they struggle every day.

The ADA has three critical roles in clinical research. The first is advocacy. The ADA advocates not only for increased dollars for NIH and CDC but also for increased access to care for people with diabetes. The organization wants to ensure that quality care is reimbursed, for the provider as well as the patient. Without reimbursement, quality care does not take place.

The ADA funds clinical research in four general areas. First, the organization identifies important clinical questions, important clinical trials, and federal trials. Second, it guides prospective donors to clinically important areas relevant to their funding interests. Many people with wealth are interested in discussing where they can best channel their resources. Generally, the larger the gift, the more direction the donor would like to exercise in the use of that gift. Third, the ADA identifies qualified investigators, both established and new, and funds their work in answering important questions about diabetes. Finally, the organization monitors the progress of research on diabetes. The ADA is not the "biggest player on the block," but it has a unique niche in helping to inspire and train young scientists and investigate areas that might not receive funding otherwise.

The ADA facilitates the translation of diabetes research into clinical practice through several vehicles. It conducts the largest meeting on diabetes in the world annually and provides a forum for the discussion of basic and clinical research. It conducts postgraduate courses for practicing clinicians in various cities throughout the year. It also holds clinical conferences on such topics as reducing cardiovascular mortality and morbidity in diabetes and understanding the effect of diabetes on cardiovascular disease. The ADA publishes three professional journals: one in basic science, one in clinical science, and one for allied health professionals. A fourth is a consumer publication for people with diabetes that provides information about the latest advances in pharmaceuticals, treatments, and care. The publication helps them engage in a dialogue with their physician or health care provider about what these advances mean for their treatment.

Several ADA committees play a role in clinical research. A professional practice committee develops diabetes care guidelines. The ADA has about 2,000 recognized education programs around the country in diabetes—office-based, hospital-based, and plan-based. It also has a provider recognition program, which is still in the development stage. The program recognizes providers who exercise best-practice performance measures in caring for people with diabetes.

The ADA is setting up an expert committee on the diagnosis and classification of diabetes and the role that impaired glucose tolerance plays. The incidence of diabetes is rising in epidemic proportions, and impaired glucose tolerance appears to be a growing factor. The association is currently examining several questions regarding the relationship between impaired glucose tolerance and diabetes: At what point do we diagnose diabetes? At what point do we diagnose impaired glucose tolerance? Is impaired glucose tolerance a separate disease? The answers to these questions have significant ramifications, such as potentially changing the number of persons with diabetes from about 16 to 20 million to 40 to 45 million. The association also prepares many clinical guidelines and position papers, such as the ADA clinical practice guidelines, which are used internationally. It helps support screening for type 2 diabetes and is preparing to release evidence-based principles and recommendations on nutrition. So the association plays a significant role in the Clinical Research Enterprise.

Needs from the perspective of the ADA include several issues. First, the business case needs to be made that prevention is important, but the cost benefit needs to be proven. It is commonly known that the onset of diabetes, particularly type 2, can be delayed, if not prevented, by the practice of appropriate health behaviors. Second, the business case needs to be made that diabetes care makes sense, i.e., that good-quality care will reduce future costs, not only for the private payer system but also down the line for the Medicare system. Third, there is a crying need for behavioral and outcomes research. If we could learn what behavioral interventions cause people to modify their behavior, we could make tremendous strides in treatment. Fourth, we need to know how to reach effectively those populations that are dispropor-

> The business case needs to be made that prevention is important . . . that good-quality care will reduce future costs, not only for the private payer system but also down the line for the Medicare system.
>
> —*John Graham IV*

tionately afflicted with diabetes. Investigating this question requires a great deal of money, and that investment has not been forthcoming.

Finally, to put forth a more provocative viewpoint, we are all participants in a capitalistic society. It is interesting that we do not provide incentives for people to take better care of themselves. The health benefits that employers pay are simply an extension of the compensation plan. We give incentives for making more "widgets" and for selling more products. In the workplace we give incentives for people to become more efficient but not for people to take better care of themselves. Why don't we? Why not give people tax credits for taking better care of themselves? People receive tax credits for child care. Companies receive tax credits for investing in research and development. Why not give people tax credits for taking care of their health? The long-term payoff might be a significant step forward.

PRIORITY SETTING IN BASIC AND CLINICAL RESEARCH

Robert Califf, M.D.
Division of Cardiology, Department of Medicine
Duke University

It is remarkable how unified the key messages were in the first part of this workshop. For all the doom and gloom projected, we need to consider that people are actually living longer and feeling better than ever. The rate of improvement, not just in survival but in disability-free survival, is growing at nearly an exponential rate in this country. Although we have identified the key diseases and causes of disability, in terms of morbidity and mortality, to be dealt with, we still have concern that the efforts of the research community are misaligned relative to the priorities of purchasers and payers.

This morning's panelists brought up the need for comparative evaluative research. Almost none of that type of research is being conducted. Why is this so, and what can be done about it? It should be remembered that the randomized clinical trial is only about 50 years old. Today's technology, with its history of only a decade or so, has made randomized clinical trials possible in a way that did not exist in earlier decades. Randomization of large numbers of subjects, and collection of pertinent data, is simple now. With technology no longer a limitation, the research structure has to catch up.

Two research models exist for conducting research: the new and the old. The old model is the so-called basic research model. It is hypothesis-driven and investigator-driven. It involves people chasing ideas in a "selfish" way, which is a good thing for basic research and is the only way to do it The largest pharmaceutical companies in the world, which invest $4 billion or $5 billion in research, are realizing that it does not work well to simply tell scientists: "We will put you at a desk and your work will be to discover a treatment for diseases A, B, and C."

Basic science works by people pursuing their curiosity. Under these conditions all kinds of interesting things happen.

The new model is evaluative research, which is entirely different. Evaluative research depends on a good structure, and the research priorities should not be set by individuals but by those who understand the health care priorities. When we confuse one model with the other, we end up with a mess on both sides. Telling basic scientists how to do their research does not work well. Turning evaluative research loose to hypothesis-driven mechanistic research produces research that is not aligned with our priorities for health care. One nuance is that research on the methodology of conducting evaluative research is basic research and should be hypothesis-driven. This type of research appears to be completely unfunded in this country.

> Evaluative research depends on a good structure, and the research priorities should be set . . . by those who understand the health care priorities.
>
> —*Robert Califf*

A reason that not many researchers are conducting evaluative research is that there is great difficulty sustaining a career in it. There is no sustained funding for this kind of work. Everyone shares in the blame for the deficiencies in our research structure. Those who train practitioners—medical schools, nursing schools—are way behind in research training. Medical students and nursing students are not being trained in how to function in a collaborative, evidence-driven environment. Medical students still spend two years in basic sciences and two years in clinical apprenticeships. If you make rounds today in most of our medical schools and ask why a certain treatment is being used, you will hear a mechanistic answer, despite the fact that we do not know the exact mechanism by which most of the highly effective treatments work.

The last thing that medical products companies want to do is comparative research. At the last count, there were 80,000 sales representatives in the U.S.A. Choosing to turn to a sales force rather than putting a product to the test is quite reasonable from a business perspective. It is just not necessarily good for the public health. One point regarding government: the government has a good policy on clinical trials coverage, but that policy is not being enforced, and the elderly are having trouble participating in clinical trials as a consequence. This problem is solvable, and the government needs to step in.

The role of the press needs to be part of the research agenda in this country. The power of the press is enormous today, and people in the research community are afraid to deal with the press. They are afraid to study the actions of the press for fear that criticism may make the press turn on them. The least of the problem is the patients. We have no trouble getting people to volunteer for clinical trials. Nearly all people who participate in clinical trials are delighted to be part of the studies, and their feedback is almost uniformly positive.

In conclusion, we have a fragmented model for the kind of research being considered today, and it needs to be put together. If the NIH, with all its resources, channeled money into an infrastructure that could leverage the participation of the payers and the medical products companies and identify top research priorities, comparative evaluative clinical research could be performed. When it is performed for reasons that are forced, such as comparing TPA with streptokinase or other easily citable models, it is effective. If we spend some money building an infrastructure within the current funding limits, and we create a model where people work together—not through hypothesis-driven models, but by identifying priorities and then putting the infrastructure to work (the NCI is close but has not yet reached this point)—we can do much to solve the problems that have been brought up today.

PRIORITY SETTING IN HEALTH SERVICES RESEARCH

Dennis Scanlon, Ph.D.
Associate Professor, Health Policy and Administration
Pennsylvania State University

> The U.S. health care system might harm patients, or even kill patients, and is not living up to its potential.
>
> —Dennis Scanlon

Two recent reports issued by the Institute of Medicine's Committee on Quality of Health Care in America, *To Err Is Human: Building a Safer Health Care System* (2001) *and Crossing the Quality Chasm: A New Health System for the 21st Century* (2001), suggest some serious problems in quality in health care in the U.S.A. The U.S. health care system might harm patients, or even kill patients, and is not living up to its potential. This realization comes at a time when health care premiums for employers and purchasers are predicted to rise by about 13% in the next year, and there is no downward trend in sight[1].

To illustrate the magnitude of those concerns, a report in an unpublished study by the Midwest Business Group on Health and the Juran Institute estimated that the direct cost of poor quality and medical errors is $1,800 per employee per year, while the indirect costs, which include lost work days and productivity, are $500 per year for a worker with an average salary of about $32,000.[2] These costs create a serious situation for those who purchase care and those who provide care. We must ask ourselves, why is there poor quality? The Institute of

---

[1] Gabel J et al. "Job-Based Health Insurance in 2001. Inflation Hits Double Digits, Managed Care Retreats" *Health Affairs*, 20(5): 180-86.

[2] Mortimer, J. "Reducing Poor Quality Care and Related Costs." March 2001. Presentation slides prepared by the President of the Midwest Business Group on Health.

Medicine reports provide insight, stating that many barriers are not the result of the incompetence of providers or inferior technical skills, but are due instead to lack of well-integrated and coordinated systems and processes for delivering health care to patients.

We still live in a paper world in health care. That reality creates the probability of errors, problems, and diminished continuity and coordination of care, which translate into poorer quality. The increasing rate of scientific development makes the cognitive decision-making task of providers much more difficult than years ago. Tools may exist for assisting providers in making decisions and helping patients make decisions that meet their preferences. However, our understanding of the impact of various interventions for coordinating patient care, improving quality, and eliminating waste and medical errors is still in its infancy. The evaluation of various interventions toward these ends, including alternative organizational and financing arrangements, should be a high priority for the Clinical Research Enterprise. Purchasers, payers, and researchers all have a role in this endeavor. In many cases the effort involves creating systems and changing culture. The irony is that at the same time that we consider these factors as potential solutions, the health insurance market is moving in the opposite direction, away from systems and away from creating organizational culture.

> We still live in a paper world in health care. That reality creates the probability of errors, problems, and diminished continuity and coordination of care, which translate into poorer quality.
>
> —Dennis Scanlon

The fastest growing form of health insurance is the preferred provider organizations (PPO). There is a move toward having employers and purchasers more or less absolve themselves from purchasing decisions and shifting these decisions to the individual consumer level. That situation is somewhat ironic. In considering additional areas for research, we see clearly that the goal from a purchaser perspective and an employer perspective is to focus on cost, health outcomes, satisfaction, and labor market outcomes. Some of those factors are easier to measure than others. For example, costs are no doubt easier to measure than health outcomes, including health status, morbidity, and mortality. The labor market outcomes such as workplace productivity are very difficult to measure. A trend for health care purchasers is the use of so-called "value-based purchasing," where they are involved in either working with or—as some might describe it—working against plans or providers in some cases to help drive the quality improvement process.

We need to understand whether partnerships between plans and purchasers, or between providers and purchasers, might lead to quality improvement. An example comes from some data presented by Dr. Ron Kessler of Harvard University in a recent paper. Dr. Kessler's study examined the prevalence of chronic conditions in employees and the relationship between these conditions and work impairment and disability days. This research is important because purchasers and employers are particularly interested in workplace productivity. Indeed, there might a place for research that attempts to link health status with productivity and to understand the relationship between the two. Programs might be developed that would help to improve not only health status but also workplace productivity.

> Researchers can assist the progress of the Clinical Research Enterprise by working with purchasers and health plans to evaluate the impact of activities, collaborative programs, and interventions.
> —Dennis Scanlon

As the recipients of health care dollars, health care providers—including health plans, hospitals, and physicians—play a prominent role in the allocation of health care resources and the quality of care received for those dollars. Research is needed on how providers can partner with purchasers to achieve creatively the objectives outlined in Dr. Kessler's research. Improving quality of care requires measurement, action, improvement, and remeasurement. This concept is demonstrated by Don Berwick's work in the Institute for Health Care. To improve quality, we need to educate providers and organizations, and we need to develop systems for engaging in measurement, acting on that measurement, and translating action into improvement.[3,4] What is the role of researchers in this process? Researchers can assist the progress of the Clinical Research Enterprise by working with purchasers and health plans to evaluate the impact of activities, collaborative programs, and interventions. Not only do we need traditional researchers with experience in conducting clinical trials, but we also need health services and social science researchers for this effort.

Many programs that require evaluation are in real-world settings, for example, as part of employment-based benefit programs or government-sponsored health insurance. In these cases, analytic techniques may be needed to account for nonrandom sample selection. Unlike typical patient trials, many of the creative interventions must involve changes in organizational structure and the use of contractual incentives, requiring the expertise of social science-based research.

Specific examples of research suggestions include the following:.

- Studies that demonstrate effective techniques for improved quality and value, including the reduction of waste and medical errors
- Studies that evaluate the potential synergy between improved health sta-

---

[3] Scanlong DP et al. "Are Managed Care Plans Organizing for Quality, "*Medical Care Research and Review*2000; 57(supplement 2), 9-32.

[4] Scanlon DP et al. "Use of Performance Measures for Improving Quality in Managed Care Organizations." *Health Services Research* 2001; 36(3): 619-641.

tus and workplace productivity, including creative interventions for achieving these goals

- Studies that demonstrate the cost-effectiveness or return-on-investment of population health interventions, including comprehensive disease management programs and that identify effective incentives for encouraging and differentially compensating high-quality care
- Studies that view employees and dependents of employer-based purchasers as populations to be studied over time
- Research that focuses on medical education training, including studies that evaluate or design mechanisms for training physicians and other clinicians to practice evidence-based medicine and to evaluate not just the effectiveness but also the cost effectiveness of treatments, and also the ability to synthesize scientific findings and incorporate their meaning into practice.

Lawrence E. Shulman, M.D., Ph.D.
Director Emeritus
National Institutes of Health

Selecting research priorities presents an enormous challenge and raises important questions. The first is, who will determine these priorities? Just the "selfish" applicant, as Dr. Califf said, or participants in consensus conferences? A second set of questions involves the burden of disease. What aspect is most important —mortality or morbidity? Which diseases are most important? Do we choose to study cancer over arthritis or aging or whatever? We have to make those particular choices. A third issue is the huge amount of data that are needed for setting public policy, for administration, and for other types of decision making. A fourth challenge is setting priorities according to the type of clinical research to be conducted. The definition of clinical research worked out at the Graylyn summit exercise (AAMC, 1999), for example, has nine different categories. We need to select priorities not only among these categories but also within each one, and this task poses difficulties. How do we choose, for instance, between therapy on the one hand and prevention on the other? Or between translational research and health services research?

Taking the broadened outlook of one who was more or less freed by semi-retirement, Dr. Shulman stated that all these things are good. He noted, for example, that all nine categories were mentioned in the talk on combating diabetes.

HEALTH SERVICES RESEARCH IN VOLUNTARY HEALTH ASSOCIATIONS

Mary Woolley of Research!America began a discussion of the health services research conducted by voluntary health associations by responding to the list of needs presented by John Graham of the ADA, which largely involve performing more behavioral and outcomes research. She asked if she was correct in assuming that, in the ADA's venture capital mode of funding research, the association addressed some of the needs that John Graham laid out. She suggested that this approach could be promoted more vigorously so that even more dollars flow into those important areas.

Enriqueta Bond of the Burroughs-Wellcome Fund asked whether the voluntary organizations are also viewing the emerging area of health services research as a major need for advancing the management of particular chronic diseases, and whether they are also advocating for dollars in this area. Has this area been a focus in the past? Might it be a larger one in the future?

John Graham replied that the ADA has become involved in outcomes research and has found some synergistic relationships. For example, the association is working with Pacificare in examining the effect of the presence of a nurse case manager in a wide diabetes practice on outcomes for people with diabetes in that practice. Outcomes research is very expensive and also very long term. It is not as glamorous as basic science. Providing a critical mass of funding that will attract researchers who will answer important questions about behavior and outcomes should considerably enhance the treatment of people with chronic disease.

> Providing a critical mass of funding that will attract researchers who will answer important questions about behavior and outcome should considerably enhance the treatment of people with chronic disease.
>
> —John Graham IV

John Graham said that the ADA has a very simple message and admitted that the association has not perfected it and could use help in getting it out. Myron Genel of Yale University suggested that the message should be simply that we need to find out what works, because that is the only way people understand health services research. He also reiterated that truly good evaluative science is expensive and requires long-term research. He lamented that as a nation we are not providing anywhere near the money needed for this type of research.

Outcomes and health services research is also an area of focus for the American Cancer Society, stated John Stevens of the ACS. He noted that the society is shifting its portfolio so that it devotes 50% of its research funding to basic research, because understanding the fundamentals of most diseases is the key to dealing with them in the long run. The other 50% is for applied research, which ranges from pre-clinical or translational research to psychosocial, behavioral, prevention, cancer control, community projects, health services, and outcomes.

An important question for the ACS is, how do you change the behavior of health care providers? Historically, one means of change has been patients' demand for a particular type of care from their physicians. Patient advocacy is one reason that mammography and the pap smear have become widespread in most segments of the population in this country. These examples demonstrate the importance of patient education in driving behavioral change in health care providers. Pharmaceutical companies are very successful at this approach through television advertising. Advertisements appear for every new product, and soon thereafter the physicians begin writing prescriptions. Either the physicians are influenced directly by the advertisements, or the patients ask for the products.

Another issue brought out by John Stevens is reimbursement of the health care provider's time for the efforts taken to provide behavioral or preventive messages. In some cases specific reimbursement is not provided for counseling against a negative health behavior. The problem then is, why would physicians spend much time providing that counseling if they know they will not be reimbursed? Unless there is reimbursement, it is very difficult to implement a procedure.

THE ROLE OF THE DEVICE INDUSTRY IN THE CLINICAL RESEARCH ENTERPRISE

Susan Foote, J.D.
Board Member
Medical Technology Leadership Forum

The Medical Technology Leadership Forum is a medical technology think tank that brings together a broad range of representatives from what is called the medical technology community, which includes physician organizations, university and research centers, health plans, device firms, bioengineering organizations, and patient groups. While the leaders from the various member organizations may have different perspectives and different incentives, they share a common goal—to contribute to public policy solutions to issues of concern to the medical technology community. This model is commendable because bringing together people who are well-meaning and involved in parts of a particular problem leads to creative thinking.

It is critical that the other participants in the Clinical Research Enterprise understand and appreciate the unique characteristics of the medical device industry and the innovative products that the industry produces. The notion that there is a distinction between engineered technologies, drug technologies, and procedures is becoming blurred in light of the innovations in genomics and new biology and in information technology applications for therapies. The device industry is a completely different industry than it was just 5 or 10 years ago.

The cost of investing in clinical trials is an important issue with many confounding viewpoints. On one hand, it is argued that the device industry should pay for the research because device firms recover the value of the investment in clinical trials when they sell the products. On the other hand, many on the side of the device industry argue that the differences between drugs and devices need to be considered:

- Devices are more dependent on physician/operator skills than most drugs.
- Innovation in devices is highly iterative, with accumulation of smaller innovations as distinct from unique chemical compounds.
- Product life cycles can be very short (18 months), and patents often confer little protection from competition.
- Clinical trial costs vary, and can be very high for some devices being studied (e.g., implanted defibrillator, artificial organ), and may cost many thousands per unit as opposed to the cost of one pill.
- Although there are many large device firms (e.g., Medtronic, St. Jude Medical, Siemens, General Electric), 80% of the firms are very small.

> If a drug or device company invests in clinical trials to obtain evidence for either the payers or the FDA, others tend to discredit those trials just because they are industry-funded.
>
> —Susan Foote

A Catch-22 in funding is an important issue in industry's investing in clinical trials. If a drug or device company invests in clinical trials to obtain evidence for either the payers or the FDA, others tend to discredit those trials just because they are industry-funded. The incentive for industry to fund the trials is to obtain data so that the approval required to sell the product will be forthcoming. The catch is, if those studies are biased, who will fund the studies and provide the information? Why can we not provide the right incentives, or design the right forums, so that industry performs studies that meet the test? Millions, maybe billions, of dollars are invested in trials sponsored by the product producers. If that money is being wasted –that is, if many of the studies are flawed—we have a problem, and it does not involve more resources. Instead, it involves trying to deploy our resources in a more constructive way in order to get value for that investment.

Other issues are timing-based. We are challenged on the device side because of the incremental nature of engineered innovations; i.e., the product life cycle of many innovations is very short and getting shorter. The short product life cycle of our own computers, for instance, helps us understand the problem facing the device industry. Considering the rapid advancement in technology, how long can you wait, or should you wait, for the trials, data, and development that are generated on a much slower time schedule than the innovation cycle of 12 to 15 months for a product?

There are structural issues, too, such as concern about conflict of interest. As the device industry and the drug industry have worked more closely with universities, there is interest from the private sector and government to redesign the conflict-of-interest rules. The Medical Technology Leadership Forum is not clear yet about how those rules should evolve. Nevertheless, the rules could pose an enormous barrier unless they are carefully drawn.

Issues of evaluation tie in to the costs of clinical trials and their credibility. What criteria do that the payers want in order to evaluate a new technology?

What standards of evidence are appropriate, and what does it mean to evaluate a study? It is difficult to have a coherent context in which to review the benefits of a new technology when the standards of evaluation are evolving as rapidly as the technology. The industry itself, in the aggregate, has some responsibility for the problems in the environment of evaluation. The politics of Medicare coverage have been intense for more than 25 years. Speaking from a medical technology perspective, we do not have a clear sense of what standards must be met. In the absence of clear standards, well-meaning people will invest a great deal of money to obtain a great deal of data that will not be well received, and none of us is well served by that situation.

THE ROLE OF THE AGENCY FOR HEALTHCARE RESEARCH AND QUALITY IN THE CLINICAL RESEARCH ENTERPRISE

Francis Chesley, M.D.
Director
Office of Research, Review, Education and Policy
Agency for Healthcare Research and Quality

The mission of the Agency for Healthcare Research and Quality (AHRQ) is to support and conduct research that will improve health outcomes, quality of care, and cost and utilization of health care services. Along the spectrum of clinical research, the AHRQ is a federal funder of health services research. We heard earlier today that it would be valuable, across the funders of clinical research, to have a reasoned approach to setting priorities in clinical research. At AHRQ, we believe that two reports from the IOM—*To Err is Human: Building a Safer Health Care System* (2000) and *Crossing the Quality Chasm: A New Health System for the 21st Century* (2001)—point us in important directions, in terms of focusing clinical research on the issue of patient safety and looking at the system of care in the U.S.A. in an empirical way. The reports also force us to think about improvements in the system of care so that we deliver the best care possible to the most people.

> We believe that two reports from the IOM—To Err is Human: Building a Safer Health Care System (2000) and Crossing the Quality Chasm: A New Health System for the 21st Century (2001)—point us in important directions.
>
> —Francis Chesley

Translating research into practice is a major priority for the agency. We also need a smart and capable cadre of researchers to conduct the research that we are talking about today. We see as very important the continued funding of not just the clinical research at large, but also the research produced by the next generation of researchers—clinical health services researchers and epidemiologists. AHRQ funds research and also conducts research. An important role we play is

> An important role we play is that of brokers—brokers of collaborations and partnerships, both public and private.
>
> —Francis Chesley

that of brokers—brokers of collaborations and partnerships, both public and private. The Evidence-based Practice Centers are one example. The National Guideline Clearinghouse, where we work with the American Medical Association and the American Association of Health Plans, is another. The issue of many clinical guidelines on the same topic is what drove the agency to seek out and work with partners.

We focused some of our research on the basis of the IOM report *To Err is Human: Building a Safer Health System* (2000). Last year, patient safety was a major focus for the agency. Researchers across the country received $50 million to examine and address issues related to patient safety. Perhaps most importantly, we looked to fund Centers of Excellence. The CERTs program is an example of a Center of Excellence that examines therapeutic agents. We have funded Centers of Excellence in patient safety and in training. We fund practice-based research networks in which nursing and physician networks actually do research with participants in clinical practice settings. It is that kind of research which will translate more broadly. We also focus on issues of health care disparity in terms of both outcome and delivery of care. The researchers are probably not the best ones to disseminate the results of that research. They probably do not receive funding for dissemination, and it may not be a priority for them. We do know, from research, what kind of mechanisms work best for disseminating information. We know from the pharmaceutical industry that there are effective ways to disseminate information to practitioners. It is fair to say that these methods do work in certain settings. Learning from that example, and figuring out how to be smart about disseminating information to those who need it —individuals as well as systems— is a need that might emerge from our introspection into the Clinical Research Enterprise.

TRANSLATIONAL BLOCKS AND PRACTICE GUIDELINES

Participants launched into a discussion of practice guidelines and their role in translating clinical research into practice. Elaine Larson of Columbia University School of Nursing started the discussion by emphasizing the importance of clinical practice guidelines as a mechanism or model for translating basic, and then applied, research into clinical practice. The National Guideline Clearinghouse has well over 1,000 clinical practice guidelines. For seven years, Larson has chaired the committee for CDC that

> There is very little external validity, i.e., little evidence as to how well these guidelines will work when widely applied nationally or globally.
>
> —Elaine Larson

writes the practice guidelines for infection prevention in health care facilities in the U.S.A. The committee has struggled during the entire seven years with how to assess the impact of the guidelines. Although the guidelines are very rigorously written and are based on randomized clinical trials and good epidemiological data, there is very little external validity, i.e., little evidence as to how well these guidelines will work when widely applied nationally or globally. The committee will soon issue a new guideline that will revolutionize certain aspects of infection control. A tremendous cultural change and much systems work will be needed to change practice, attitudes, and values. Elaine Larson warned that we are not prepared for that kind of research. We are prepared in terms of how the research should be done but not in terms of how to get people to change.

When we talk to institutions about partnering with us in assessing impact, we are told that they have only a small role in that endeavor. To reiterate a question asked earlier, how do we transform the research and professional culture into a team sport? Those of us in the Clinical Research Roundtable need to get beyond the rhetoric about being a team and take action to determine what kinds of efforts, recommendations, practices, and perhaps research at the systems level are needed to bring about that team culture.

Robert Califf of Duke University mentioned that every practitioner knows that the current guidelines apply to only a small part of his or her everyday professional life. In cardiology we have solid evidence for a few factors that affect major outcomes. There is a very nice correlation between mortality rates and guideline compliance. The most important elements of the guidelines could be pared down to perhaps 10 processes of care for which there is good evidence of a relationship between process and outcome. Actually, probably fewer than 10 are broadly applicable to almost everything we do.

John Graham of the ADA noted that attaining the culture of a team sport is very difficult and requires a paradigm shift. He pointed out that certain disorders and diseases need to be treated in an acute manner that lends itself to the "cowboy mentality," and that this mentality might even be preferred in treating those diseases. Other, more chronic, diseases such as arthritis and diabetes lend themselves to ongoing management. Although not every individual responds in the same way to care, in diabetes care following certain performance measures leads to certain outcomes. Health systems and employers need to be willing to pay the costs and should require the implementation and enforcement of that kind of system.

> We have not figured out, however, how to measure the impact of the reports and other documents on clinical care.
>
> *—Francis Chesley*

Francis Chesley of the AHRQ stated that the AHRQ has evolved away from traditional guidelines and toward evidence reports, in the scheme of what is actually an evidence-based practice approach to clinical medicine. AHRQ will not do research unless it has a partner, public or private, to address three or four key questions that will inform their clinical practice or their approach to clinical practice. If there is no evidence to answer those questions (and often there is not), the process is stopped. The evidence report is not a clinical practice guideline; instead, it represents a start for an organization or a group of practitioners who are federal partners, who then take the answers to those questions and move that knowledge into their practice environment. At AHRQ we have learned that if the creation of the document does not involve persons who are likely to use it once completed, there is less likelihood that the document will have any real impact. We have not figured out, however, how to measure the impact of the reports and other documents on clinical care. One focus for the agency this year will be to fund research that examines how to translate research into practice and measure the impact of that work.

SUMMARY

The goal of the session on the role of other stakeholders in the Clinical Research Enterprise was to examine how voluntary health associations, academic institutions, research organizations, and the medical device industry contribute to the Clinical Research Enterprise and what they need from the enterprise to better promote health and health care (see box).

Representatives from voluntary health organizations (the American Cancer Society and the American Diabetes Association) stated the mission of their organizations, described their research and advocacy efforts, and discussed their educational programs for professionals, patients, and the public. Representatives from academic institutions (Duke University and Pennsylvania State University) spoke about the emergence of evaluative research, which moves away from individual, hypothesis-driven basic research toward collaborative research with a social science base. A former Institute director from the National Institutes of Health pointed out the challenges involved in setting research priorities nationally. A representative from the Medical Technology Leadership Forum emphasized the unique characteristics of the medical device industry and the challenges the industry faces in funding research, obtaining timely research results, and evaluating those results. A representative from the Agency for Healthcare Research and Quality described the mission of the agency and spoke about its role as a broker of public and private collaborations and partnerships. Finally, participants discussed the need for a paradigm shift that would transform the current research and professional culture into a team effort.

Highlights of Session on the Role of Other Stakeholders in the Clinical Research Enterprise

What can voluntary health associations, academic institutions, research organizations, and the medical device industry contribute to the Clinical Research Enterprise?

- Voluntary health associations such as the American Cancer Society and the American Diabetes Association contribute to the Clinical Research Enterprise by participating in and funding clinical research; recruiting patients for trials; advocating for funding and for high-quality patient care; translating research into clinical practice; educating professionals, patients, and the public; and in assisting in the creation of clinical guidelines.
- The medical device industry produces innovative products that contribute to the armamentarium of health care treatments. Leaders of the medical technology community share the common goal of contributing to public policy solutions to issues of concern in that community.
- The Agency for Healthcare Research and Quality supports and conducts research that will improve health outcomes, quality of care, and cost and utilization of health care services. Translating research into practice is a main priority. An important role is that of brokers of collaborations and partnerships—both public and private.

What do these organizations need from the Clinical Research Enterprise to better promote health and health care?

- The results of basic research through the Clinical Research Enterprise have been critical to progress in the prevention and treatment of diseases such as cancer and diabetes, but more research is needed.
- The business case needs to be made that disease prevention is important; i.e., the cost benefit of preventive methods needs to be proven.
- Consumers need to be given incentives to take better care of their health.
- Barriers to the dissemination of research and clinical information need to be eliminated. Protection of privacy is also essential, particularly in light of rapid progress in genome research.
- An infrastructure must be put in place for a new type of research—evaluative research—that is aligned with overall priorities for health care.
- Interventions for coordinating patient care, improving quality, and eliminating waste and medical errors should be evaluated. All stakeholders have a role in this endeavor, which will involve creating systems and changing the existing health care culture.
- Research is needed on how partnerships among providers, purchasers, and payers can create quality improvement in health care delivery.
- Selecting clinical research priorities poses an enormous challenge but must be attempted. Questions include: Who should determine these priorities? What aspects of selected diseases warrant the most attention? What type of clinical research needs to be conducted?
- A "Catch-22" in funding of research by industry needs to be resolved. Research findings may be discredited when industry invests in clinical trials to obtain evidence for payers or the FDA; yet who else will fund the research and provide the information? More guidance is needed as to how to evaluate research findings and what standards must be met.
- The Clinical Research Enterprise needs to promote a paradigm shift that would transform the current individual-driven research and professional culture into a team effort.

4

Opportunities and Challenges in the Clinical Research Enterprise

INTRODUCTION

Allan Korn, M.D.
Workshop Co-Chair
Senior Vice President and Chief Medical Officer
Blue Cross Blue Shield Association

All the cowboys and all the cows go in one direction. Why do they do that? It is because when they get to Abilene, they get paid. There is a lesson there. The Clinical Research Enterprise faces the challenge of driving the current system toward high quality care. The Enterprise is made up of diverse stakeholders with vested yet often conflicting interests. To make the necessary improvements, cooperation must be cast as tangible benefits for each of these stakeholders. This poses another obstacle however, as conflict of interest may cause doubt about the integrity of those who stand to gain too much from a particular outcome. Studies are done by groups who have an incentive to ask a certain question. It is recognized that a particular member may not ask the "right" question from the view of the overall enterprise. As a group, we need to figure out how to incent the individual members of the Clinical Research Enterprise to ask the questions that need to be answered and move beyond the second translational block from clinical knowledge to practice. Moreover, how do you create incentives in such a way that they do not exacerbate conflicts of interest, and/or mitigate those that already exist. The cowboys and cows go to Abilene because they have an incentive to do so. We need to create a similar pull in clinical research today.

Next we are going to hear from Lou Sherwood from Merck and Co. about disease management and the importance of outcomes research. Myrl Weinberg will also discuss the idea of integrated patient-centered care. There is a changing relationship between patients and their healthcare providers that necessitates a more integral role for patients at every step of the decision making process. This is just one of many things that must be considered when rethinking the process by which health care decisions are made and implemented so as to improve the health of the country.

OUTCOMES RESEARCH AND DISEASE MANAGEMENT

Lou Sherwood, M.D.
Senior Vice President for Medical and Scientific Affairs
Merck and Company

The second frontier is getting physicians to practice evidence-based medicine (setting care objectives, collecting data, and being accountable for the results). We need a great deal of additional research to figure out how to do all of this optimally. The thousands of Continuing Medical Education lectures delivered every year in academic institutions and by the pharmaceutical industry do not accomplish the goal of reaching the second frontier. That goal involves starting with outcomes research and moving to disease management. Outcomes research examines the consequences of medical treatment that are noticeable to patients and their families. It includes typical dichotomous variables, such as whether people live or die, and the so-called humanistic outcomes such as quality of life, functional status, and patient satisfaction—things that are vitally important to patients and their families. The third variable is the associated costs.

> The thousands of Continuing Medical Education lectures delivered every year in academic institutions and by the pharmaceutical industry do not accomplish the goal of reaching the second frontier.
>
> —*Lou Sherwood*

Why do we want to measure outcomes? It is important to do so because people are beginning to look critically and measure what various products and their organizations do in relation to health care. In light of the consolidation of health care and the changes being made, it is critically important that these measures be examined. We must have a structure, look at process, measure outcomes, and try to continually improve what we do.

What is meant by structure, process, and outcome? If patients' risk factors are not being addressed in a secondary prevention mode (the things that we know work), we are not delivering quality care, and patients are not receiving the benefits of the research conducted over several decades. Movement from outcomes research to outcomes management or disease management occurs when one seeks to produce desirable outcomes in usual clinical settings. It involves marrying the practice of medicine with the principles of public health.

> We need to move the paradigm ahead. In an informatics era it is unacceptable for physicians not to be tuned in to the advances in medicine and not to be implementing them in their practices.
>
> —Lou Sherwood

Physicians will continue to deliver care to one patient at a time, but they must start collecting data across their populations of patients. It would be useful if the average pediatrician had a data base on all immunizations of the children in his or her practice. It would also be useful if the primary care physician who, on average, has 1,200 or 1,300 post-menopausal women in his or her practice had a database on their pap smear results and mammograms, as well as assessment of cardiovascular, osteoporosis, and mental health risks. We need to move the paradigm ahead because in an information era it is unacceptable and borders on the unethical for physicians not to be tuned in to the advances in medicine and not to be implementing them in their practices. Major changes in information systems and infrastructure are needed to help physicians achieve those goals.

Disease management is a process that assists payers and providers in improving clinical outcomes and quality of life, and in managing health care costs using the principles of quality management. What is needed is an infrastructure and a common set of outcome measures that are endorsed by providers. If guidelines are "shrink-wrapped on someone's shelf," they do no good. What is essential is that at the local level, in the medical group, practitioners must adopt a guideline—either their own or someone else's—with an eye toward process. This process entails setting objectives, collecting data, and looking at what happens to people.

The problem is that we do not know how to perform this form of applied clinical research well. A major barrier is not just the lack of a universal electronic medical record, or the absence of an infrastructure, but the mindset of physicians. Physicians have had limited training and orientation to this way of thinking. Not only must we teach the students, but we also have to train the faculty. We train physicians to be independent thinkers, and that is commendable. But if they cannot block and tackle, who would want them on their football team? Imagine eleven independent thinkers running around the field! Teamwork is essential, and it is something we learn about in industry.

In medical practice, there is heterogeneity well beyond what the data support, and we know that the variation is related to different outcomes. The critical question that we have considered in today's workshop is, how do we institute systems of care that improve outcomes for a population? This is not to say that every patient should be treated in exactly the same way; yet certain common themes emerge that ensure optimal care if data are collected across all patients for common diseases. Again, modern information systems are critical for achieving this aim.

We must start thinking about managing the total cost of health care, not just individual cost centers. We tend to work in a "silo mentality," where each segment of the organization focuses on its own budget, when these budgets are actually closely linked. The Department of Veterans Affairs, for example, in setting up an effective system to connect various segments of the department, has been a pioneer this area.

We have published studies containing findings taken from the records of about 50,000 patients with coronary heart diseases; these records were drawn from the practices of several hundred cardiologists.[1] The findings were appalling, even in terms of accomplishing cholesterol screening, much less in achieving the outlined goals. In a follow-up study, 10 groups of cardiologists met to define the objectives for patients with coronary heart disease. They did have a common set of objectives, however, and they had to collect a common data set. The only common variable among the groups that did the best work was the presence of a nurse or nurse practitioner who made sure that the work was done, that the patients received the right care, and that patients' risk factors were addressed.[2] The study pointed to the need for stronger research efforts. Physicians have to drive the quality of care, but they also have to control the costs.

The old paradigm of a condescending flow of information from physician to patient no longer holds. The new paradigm is a dynamic relationship in which information is shared and the physician, appropriately informed, can present choices to patients and families, who can then make informed decisions. The key is to maximize provider resources and expertise, with the help of systems, but maintain a true partnership between physician and patient.

> The new paradigm is a dynamic relationship in which information is shared and the physician, appropriately informed, can present choices to patients, who can then make informed decisions.
>
> —Lou Sherwood

How do you change behavior? By setting objectives and goals and using

---

[1] Sueta CA, Chowdhury M, Boccuzzi SJ, Smith SC, Alexander CM, Londhe A, Lulla A, Simpson RJ. Analysis of the Degree of Undertreatment of Hyperlipidemia and Congestive Heart Failure Secondary to Coronary Artery Disease. Am J Cardiol. 1999; 83: 1303-1307.

[2] Walsh MN, Wan GJ, Kuo LC, Eisenberg DA, Simposn RJ, Pearson TA, Alexander CM. Application of disease management principles to achieve national guideline-defined goals for patients with coronary heart disease. Journal of General Internal Medicine 2000; 15 (Suppl 1): 153. Presented at SGIM Annual Meeting, Boston, MA May 2000.

quality measures, by examining one's own data, benchmarking, and systems support. Carrots are nice, but sometimes sticks are necessary. Our traditional educational programs, whether medical school curricula or other areas, are grossly inadequate. We must experiment in this arena, because we are remarkably short on knowledge of how to change behavior.

Merck recently sponsored a major observational study called NORA the one year follow-up study of a cohort of 200,000 women.[3] The background for this study was the magnitude of the burden of osteoporotic fractures and the fact that bone density measurements have been shown to predict fracture risks, along with other risk factors. The study objectives were to report the occurrence of low bone mass in a large cohort of ethnically diverse post-menopausal women, examine the relationships between bone density and fractures, and relate other risk factors to fracture risk.

From September 1997 to March 1999, 200,000 women were randomly selected at 4,100 primary care offices. At baseline these women had a mean age of about 65 years. In this population, nearly half had low bone mass. Seven percent had frank osteoporosis according to the World Health Organization criteria. Forty percent had so-called osteopenia, i.e., their bone density reading was −1 to −2.5 (1 to 2.5 standard deviations below the mean). Sixty-three percent of the women had taken estrogen.

Those women who were currently taking estrogen had a higher bone density; those who had been taking it for 10 years or more had the highest bone density. Women who had taken estrogen for even 10 years or more had lost most or all of the bone density they had previously gained if they had discontinued taking it for 5 years or more. Within the one-year follow-up period, 1.5% of the women sustained fractures. When we looked at the bone density by cohorts, we found that the women with the lowest bone density had the highest likelihood of having fractures. Using a baseline questionnaire and an inexpensive bone density test, we were able to predict quite accurately the women in this cohort who would have fractures. Regardless of what instrument we used, the findings were essentially the same. The cohort continues to be followed and the two year data will be available soon. This is the largest cohort of post-menopausal women being followed in an observational study.

We have been experimenting with guidelines and pathways, but we really need to move to document outcomes and have physicians and others make measurements and be accountable. The real question is, how long will it take? We need providers, payers, and patients to increase their sophistica-

---

[3] Siris ES, Miller PD, Barrett-Connor E, Faulkner KG, Wehren LE, Abbott TA, Berger ML, Santora AC, Sherwood LM. Identification of fracture outcomes of undiagnosed low bone mineral density in postmenopausal women. Results from the National Osteoporosis Risk Assessment. JAMA, Dec 12,, 2001; Col. 286, No. 22: 2815-2822.

tion so that they understand this new way to think about and practice medicine. We need to develop methods to resolve long-standing issues that have presented barriers to evidenced-based practice. These methods include changing medical school curricula, building systems and infrastructure, and orienting people in this direction.

INTEGRATED PATIENT-CENTERED CARE

Focusing the discussion on integrated approaches to patient care, Myrl Weinberg of the National Health Council described an initiative called integrated patient-centered care, which goes beyond disease management. This initiative takes into account the patient with multiple chronic diseases and looks at the whole person. It is particularly applicable to the older population. Information is shared across providers, including information that providers rarely receive about complementary and alternative treatments that people are self-managing. The question is, how does this effort fit into what has just been discussed?

The National Council on Quality Assurance is currently finalizing standards for the accreditation of disease management programs. Just as we begin to consider a more holistic, integrated, patient-centered approach to care, disease management companies are contracting with health plans to handle one disease at a time. The progression has been from viewing the patient as a body organ to viewing the patient as a disease. The Clinical Research Enterprise needs to ask the question, what kind of clinical research will guide the decisions as to what is put into practice and how practice is carried out? Otherwise, we will be performing more segmented, targeted clinical research, rather than anticipating a system that considers the whole patient.

Lou Sherwood of Merck suggested that having all the information about a patient in one place is the "holy grail" of evidence-based medicine. He noted that this approach is essential in an aging population and that it represents a new process in the delivery of care

Myron Genel of Yale University agreed that disease management is the product of clinical research and that the evaluative sciences will help guide proper decisions for improving disease management. He mentioned that efforts to change behavior are enhanced when the relationship between physician and patient is stable.

RESEARCH PRIORITIES IN PHARMACEUTICAL COMPANIES

Participants in the workshop turned to the issue of research funding, noting the many difficulties to be overcome. Sean Tunis of the Centers for Medicare and Medicaid Services began by suggesting that the osteoporosis study described earlier by Lou Sherwood of Merck and Company highlights a fundamental problem in research—conflict of interest. Researchers at Merck may not have designed the study and decided to fund it by considering what would be the most important clinical question to ask in osteoporosis prevention. Rather, Sean Tunis suggested that a study on the prevalence of osteoporosis in a huge cohort of women may have been appealing because it potentially serves the needs of a company that produces an important drug for the treatment of osteoporosis. He postulated that an important clinical question about osteoporosis prevention in women at low risk would be whether taking calcium supplements twice a day had as much effect on bone density loss as taking Fosamax.

Lou Sherwood replied that Merck did conduct a three-armed study that examined the effects of calcium supplementation. Results showed no additive effect of the calcium over and above the alendronate and little or no benefit from calcium alone. This has been well documented in the osteoporosis literature.

Sean Tunis responded that the essential issue is that the priority-setting mechanism for Merck may not be what payers want. He observed that the large osteoporosis study was supported by those who produce scans to detect low-density bone mass and by those who sell a drug to treat osteoporosis. Because we are faced with trying to figure out how to direct limited financial resources to the most important research questions, there are reasons to think that the constructive interaction of self-interest noted in the case of the osteoporosis study may not be the way that the Clinical Research Enterprise produces the most valuable knowledge for the money.

Lou Sherwood replied that Merck's incentives for the study are aligned with those of the National Osteoporosis Foundation in terms of helping to identify women who were at risk for this disease. He noted the importance of making physicians and patients aware of the advances that have taken place in osteoporosis. A main incentives for conducting the study was to help educate physicians as well as post-menopausal women. He acknowledged that the pharmaceutical company has profit incentives, but not in a way that does not enhance health. The key question is, what can we do to improve health? If a woman is diagnosed with osteoporosis, and there is a well-studied medication that is appropriate for that person, we might expect it to be used. It is a question of where the incentives are. Those who are paying for osteoporosis care may not want to deal with this issue. Fortunately, the Bone Mass Measurement Act was passed, and women covered by Medicare can now be reimbursed for bone density measurement.

Patricia Salber of General Motors Corporation noted that the osteoporosis study revealed that the number of women with clinically significant conditions related to their osteoporosis was relatively small. She raised a question as to whether all those women need Fosamax simply because, according to some guideline, their bone mineral density is considered low. Do we want to ask the question, who amongst all those people actually needs to have the treatment? The key question then becomes, who would be interested in funding a study to examine which patients have the condition but do not need the drug?

Rick Martinez of Johnson & Johnson entered the discussion by speculating that payers are experiencing growing pains, transitioning from consumers of research to potential sponsors of research. He also stressed the importance of differentiating among the kinds of research under consideration. The motivations for supporting basic research and clinical research are very different. Certainly, the motivations behind pharmaceutical-sponsored research are different from those driving government-sponsored research through NIH, which is more curiosity driven. Industry is product-driven. The question of how payers inform their unique decisions will remain unsettled until the commercial insurers and investor-owned HMO's conduct studies for their products.

William Crowley of Massachusetts General Hospital noted that the first translational level of research is largely and quantitatively funded by two groups in this country, NIH and pharmaceutical companies. Agencies such as the Veterans Administration, the Department of Education, the Department of Defense, and the Environmental Protection Agency, as well as some professional societies, do some research but in a limited role. Clinical trials are quantitatively driven by the pharmaceutical industry first, the biotechnical industry second, and now the NIH. He asked, what happens after that, at the second translational block? Although some infrastructure is in place for the first and the second groups, essentially no infrastructure is in place for the third. The cost to put it in place would be enormous, considering the information technology needed, the methodology required, the variety of community-based organizations affected, the large number of patients involved, and the breadth of disease states. The relative cost of such an effort needs to be kept in perspective.

Consider for a moment that $1.5 trillion is spent on health care in this country, and let us say that 1% is the amount to be devoted to such an effort. That is $15 billion, compared, for example, with a total annual budget for the NIH of $24 billion. We have to tie the spectrum and the quantitation together because we cannot discuss one without the other.

A paradigm shift in all types of research is that the individual, investigator-driven research is giving way, at all levels of research, to research conducted by large coalitions of multidisciplinary groups. Even the genomic research is performed by a multidisciplinary group. Those in industry have learned how to handle, encourage, and reward team research. In contrast, payers, providers, academic centers, and medical schools have almost no cultural background in using this approach. The paradigm is individual, investigator-initiated research, which is not "selfish research," but rather inquiry-driven research, without which much collateral research would not be performed. The demand from the public, the demand from the genome project, the demand from everyone at this workshop is large, multidisciplinary groups.

> Happy are the circumstances when the public health and the private wealth converge.
>
> —*Hugh Tilson*

That is what the members of the Clinical Research Roundtable are so excited about. It is the coalitions that receive funding, not individual groups, because there is such a major paradigm shift afoot.

Rick Martinez noted that more than 100,000 physicians are currently in various residency programs. Most of those physicians will finish without any exposure to research methodology and with no experience working with biostatisticians or with those who design clinical trials. The situation is unfortunate, especially given the promise of genomics. The problem, however, is not unique to medical schools; even undergraduate education silos its departments of psychology, statistics, and mathematics to operate in relative isolation from each other.

Hugh Tilson of the University of North Carolina emphasized that the ethics and politics of who pays for research should be revised often, remarking: "Happy are the circumstances when the public health and the private wealth converge." So much work needs to be done that if industry receives some gain from the research and is willing to pay for it, the effort is commendable. Hugh Tilson commended Lou Sherwood on the published article on the osteoporosis study, not just because it is a good article, but because Merck scientists are listed as authors.

As a scientist who worked in industry for 15 years, Hugh Tilson commented that he was never amused when it was suggested that he should not be listed as author of an article when he had done a great deal of the scientific work. The suggestion was made, he said, because of the perception that if he worked in industry he could not be trusted and, consequently, the content of the article could not be trusted. Conflict of interest is a difficult issue, and one that we need to keep addressing squarely at this roundtable.

> The training of epidemiologists and outcomes researchers is inadequate even for industry research, much less for the research urgently demanded by the roundtable. Nor is training adequate for accomplishing the large public health practice and systems research agenda.
>
> —Hugh Tilson

Another challenging issue is how to use the $16 billion to do what is needed on the right side of the research agenda, i.e., on the public health side. If there is funding for this effort, researchers may be drawn to the field. On the other hand, if no researchers are trained to do the work, no amount of money will bring results, at least not in the short run. The training of epidemiologists and outcomes researchers is inadequate even for industry research, much less for the research urgently demanded by the roundtable. Nor is training adequate for accomplishing the large public health practice and systems research agenda.

It is shocking that in America today no centers are funded to do public health systems research. We must close that gap if we are to have any understanding of the circumstances that cause us to be healthy, or at least the circumstances that help us forestall the otherwise inevitable, inexorable, and sometimes rapid progression from wellness to illness. We need to stop that progression at the population and environmental level, and this effort will require an enormous investment in an infrastructure that must be created from scratch.

Hugh Tilson noted that the Centers for Education and Research in Therapeutics (CERTS) are another greatly under-funded area, and he mentioned that five years ago, no centers existed for education and research into the translation of what is known about treatment into improved practices of therapeutics. Such centers might address questions that do not necessarily have the proprietary interest that would draw industry sponsorship.

Recognizing the gap in funding, Congress appropriated funds for the CERTS as part of the FDA Modernization Act. Those seven centers are now funded through AHRQ collaboratively with the FDA. Applications to AHRQ for therapeutics research must include a proposal for a program of research that improves health specifically by improving the translation of what is known into what is done therapeutically. These centers provide the opportunity to fund the capacity for the research and not just the research projects themselves. In another stroke of genius, AHRQ funded centers conditionally on something that academia has always had a difficult time doing. Does anyone want to guess what? They have to work together! Representatives from the seven centers are required to come to the table quarterly as collaborators to examine the development of cross-academic synergy. This mechanism pulls the group together in a coordinated activity chaired by a national coordinating center, directed by Robert Califf of Duke University, and a national steering committee, chaired by Hugh Tilson.

The centers were instructed to develop public-private partnerships as part of their long-term sustained viability. They were charged with creating the context in which the long-standing distrust and adversity between the private sector— the pharmaceutical industry, particularly in therapeutics—and academia and practice could be overcome. The purpose was to create a context for industry and academia to come as partners and develop research projects jointly, and to propose these projects to industry and voluntary partners for co-funding and collaborative work (including industry researchers as authors on research articles). Federal funding was to be reserved for projects for which private funding was not forthcoming. We are working hard on continued evolution and application of a set of principles for public-private partnership to ensure that all of the interests at the table can be heard, respected, and advanced.

Bill Sigmund of Pfizer stated that sometimes the misperception of industry-based research is that it is tainted and of low quality, but much effort is made to

> Clinical researchers must be trained not only in clinical research methods but also in the dissemination of the information.
>
> —Bill Sigmund

ensure quality. Clinical researchers must be trained not only in clinical research methods but also in the dissemination of the information. Patients vary in their ability to make sound health care decisions, and we need to work on developing the best ways to communicate and disseminate the information to all of them.

Concluding the session, Allan Korn posited that demand-driven medicine is effective, as demonstrated by the efforts of the American Cancer Society. On the other hand, we face an issue when, for example, patients demand bone marrow transplants that are probably more harmful than helpful; demand spiral CT scans if they have been tobacco smokers, long before the NIH reports whether or not results from these scans are meaningful; or demand spiral CT scans of the coronary arteries as screening tools rather than diagnostic aids. We want to demand the right things. One reason we exist as a roundtable is the continued pressure created by unrestrained expectations in an environment of limited resources. We have to be very careful when we open the door to the expectation that all demands can be satisfied and allow everyone through it.

SUMMARY

The purpose of the session on opportunities and challenges in the Clinical Research Enterprise was to tie together points made in early sessions of the workshop, explore opportunities for new approaches to research and patient care, and examine the challenges inherent in research funding, such as provision of incentives and conflict of interest (see box).

A representative from Merck and Company described outcomes research that can assist with disease management, citing recent research on osteoporosis prevention. A representative from the National Health Council described an initiative—integrated patient-centered care—that extends beyond disease management by taking into account the whole person, who may have multiple chronic diseases. Finally, participants discussed incentives in research funding and the conflict of interest that can result. They acknowledged a trend toward, and a need for, a paradigm shift from investigator-driven research to research conducted by large coalitions of multidisciplinary groups.

Highlights of Session on Opportunities and Challenges in the Clinical Research Enterprise

What are the opportunities for new approaches to research and patient care?

- Having physicians practice evidence-based medicine, setting care objectives, collecting data, and being accountable involves starting with outcomes research and moving to disease management.
- Outcomes research examines the consequences of medical treatment in terms of what is important to patients and their families—not only dichotomous variables such as whether people live or die, but also humanistic outcomes such as quality of life, functional status, and patient satisfaction. Such research provides a key to disease management.
- Disease management is a process that assists payers and providers in improving clinical outcomes and quality of life, and in managing health care costs using the principles of quality management.
- The total cost of health care, not just individual cost centers, must be managed. The Department of Veterans Affairs provides a model for such management.
- A new paradigm in the relationship between physician and patient is a dynamic relationship in which information is shared and the physician can present choices to the patient, who can then make informed decisions.
- Integrated patient-centered care goes beyond disease management because it takes into account the patient with multiple chronic diseases and looks at the whole person. Information is shared across providers.

What are the challenges facing the Clinical Research Enterprise?

- Methods must be developed to resolve long-standing issues that have presented barriers to evidence-based practice. These methods include changing medical school curricula, building systems and infrastructure, and orienting providers, purchasers, payers, and patients in this direction.
- The issue of how to provide payers with information that they can use to inform their decisions must be settled. Currently, investigator initiated research sponsored by the government and product-driven research supported by industry may not adequately address the information needs of the payers. Conflict-of-interest issues in funding need to be addressed.
- The paradigm shift from individual, investigator-driven research to research conducted by large coalitions of multidisciplinary groups—which is being driven by demand from public, the genome project, and all stakeholders in the Clinical Research Enterprise—will require a large infrastructure and an enormous funding effort.

Suggested Readings

Association of American Medical Colleges. 1999. *Breaking the Scientific Bottleneck; Clinical Research: A National Call to Action.* Washington, D.C.: AAMC Press.

Committee on Quality of Health Care in America, Institute of Medicine. 2000. *To Err Is Human: Building a Safer Health System.* Washington, D.C.: National Academy Press.

Committee on Quality of Health Care in America, Institute of Medicine. 2001. *Crossing the Quality Chasm: A New Health System for the 21st Century.* Washington, D.C.: National Academy Press.

Gabel J et al. "Job-Based Health Insurance in 2001. Inflation Hits Double Digits, Managed Care Retreats," *Health Affairs* 2001; 20(5): 180-186.

Mortimer J. "Reducing Poor Quality Care and Related Costs." March 2001. Presentation slides prepared by the President of the Midwest Business Group on Health.

Scanlon DP et al. "Are Managed Care Plans Organized for Quality ?" *Medical Care Research and Review* 2000; 57(supplement 2), 9-32.

Scanlon DP et al. "Use of Performance Measures for Improving Quality in Managed Care Organizations," *Health Services Research* 2001; 36(3): 619-641.

Solbert L.I., Kottke T.E., Brekke, M.L. 2001. Variation in clinical preventive services. Effective Clinical Practice 4(3):121-126.

Appendix I

Speaker Biographies

Jill Berger is the Director of Benefit Plan Quality Management for Marriott International, a leading hospitality company with 140,000 employees nationwide. Ms. Berger is responsible for the strategy, design and administration of Marriott's benefit plans—with a concentration in health plan quality improvement. Ms. Berger is an active member of the Leapfrog Group for Patient Safety, whose goal is to initiate breakthroughs in the safety and quality of healthcare. Ms. Berger is also on the Board of Directors for RxHealthValue, a coalition of purchasers, health plans and academic researchers whose goal is to develop approaches through research and legislative activities to the prescription drug challenge.

Prior to working for Marriott, Ms. Berger was with Kaiser Permanente, working in conjunction with General Motors as a Health Plan Manager. Prior to working with General Motors, Ms. Berger was manager, medical plans for Sears, Roebuck and Company who provides health benefits for over 250,000 employees and retirees. Ms. Berger obtained her Bachelor of Arts degree from Mount St. Mary's College and her MSA from Johns Hopkins University.

Eric Book, MD is Wellmark's Group Vice President and Chief Medical Officer. In his position, Dr. Book is responsible for the company's medical management activities including health improvement initiatives, benefits management, NCQA accreditation activities, and health data reporting. Prior to joining Wellmark, Dr. Book served as Chief Medical Officer for Primera Healthcare in Denver, Colorado, where he was responsible for the overall development and management of the clinical delivery system, including the development of physician governance and the management infrastructure for ambulatory health care delivery. Dr. Book, a board certified family physician, received his Doctor of Medicine in 1971 from the University of Toronto and is a member of the American College of Physician Executives, the American Medical Association, and the American Academy of Family Physicians.

Robert M. Califf, MD is currently Associate Vice Chancellor for Clinical Research, Director of the Duke Clinical Research Institute (DCRI), and Professor of Medicine, Division of Cardiology, at the Duke University Medical Center, Durham, NC. He has served as an editor for the first and second editions of the landmark textbook, *Acute Coronary Care*, published by Mosby, Inc., and is the Editor-in Chief of Mosby's *American Heart Journal*. He graduated from Duke University, *summa cum laude* and Phi Beta Kappa, in 1973 and from Duke University Medical School in 1978, where he was selected for Alpha Omega Alpha. He is board-certified in Internal Medicine (1984) and Cardiology (1986) and is a Fellow of the American College of Cardiology (1988). Dr. Califf has led the DCRI efforts for many of the best-known clinical trials in cardiovascular disease. He has served on the Cardiorenal Advisory Panel of the U.S. Food and Drug Administration (FDA). He also served on several IOM Committees. He is Director of coordinating center for the Centers for Education & Research in Therapeutics' (CERTs), a public-private partnership among the Agency for Healthcare Research and Quality, the FDA, academia, the medical products industry, and consumer groups.

Charles Cutler, MD, MS has over 20 years of experience in leadership positions in managed care. Currently, he serves as Chief Medical Officer for the American Association of Health Plans Before joining AAHP, Dr. Cutler was with Prudential HealthCare where he filled two roles as Vice President, Medical Services and President of the Prudential Center for Health Care Research. After completing a residency in Internal Medicine at the University of Minnesota Hospitals, Dr. Cutler joined Rhode Island Group Health Association, a staff model HMO. He has practiced general internal medicine, taught medical students and residents at Brown University teaching hospitals, and has assumed a range of administrative positions beginning with Chief of Internal Medicine in 1979. Dr. Cutler was a Sloan Fellow at the Sloan School of Management at MIT, earning a Master of Management Science (the Sloan equivalent of an MBA) in 1989. He has received degrees from NYU (MD 1973) and the University of Chicago (AB 1969). He is a member of the American College of Physicians, the American College of Physician Executives, the International Society for Quality in Health Care, and the International Association of Technology Assessment in Health Care.

Helen Darling is president of the Washington Business Group on Health

(WBGH). The Business Group is the nation's only non-profit organization devoted exclusively to representing large employers' perspective on national health policy issues and providing practical solutions to its members' most important health care problems. In addition to her WBGH responsibilities, Darling currently serves as co-chair of the National Committee on Quality Assurance Committee on Performance Measure, an independent non-profit association whose mission is to evaluate and report on the quality of the nation's managed care organizations. She is also a member of the Medical Advisory Panel, Technology Evaluation Center, run by the Blue Cross Blue Shield Association.

Prior to joining the Business Group, Darling served as Senior Consultant, Group Benefits and Health Costs for Watson Wyatt and Company, a global consulting firm that provides services in employee benefits and human resources. Prior to working for Watson Wyatt, Darling directed the purchasing of health benefits and disability for thousands of employees and retirees at Xerox Corporation. Darling received her master's degree in Demography/Sociology and her bachelor's of science degree in History/English, cum laude, from Memphis State University.

Susan Bartlett Foote, JD is an Associate Professor and head of the Division of Health Services Research and Policy at the University of Minnesota. She serves on the Board of the Medical Technology Leadership Forum, and has served as an advisor to the FDA, the Office of Technology Assessment (OTA), and the NIH. Prior to her arrival at Minnesota in 1999, she was a professor of business and public policy at the Haas School of Business at the University of California, Berkeley. From 1990–1994, she was a Robert Wood Johnson Health Policy Fellow and Senior Legislative Analyst in the office of Senator Dave Durenberger of Minnesota. She was a consultant on health policy issues in Washington, D.C. from 1995–1999. Her research has focused on the influences of public policies on health care services, with a particular emphasis on innovation in medical technology. She is the author of *Managing the Medical Arms Race: Innovation and Public Policy in the Medical Device Industry* as well as numerous articles on technology policy. She holds a JD degree from Boalt Hall, University of California, Berkeley.

John H. Graham IV is the Chief Executive Officer of the American Diabetes Association (ADA) in Alexandria, Virginia. ADA is the leading non-profit health organization supporting diabetes research, public, patient and professional information and advocacy. The Association has offices throughout the United States serving the 16 million people with diabetes through thousands of volunteers and over 900 staff. John has served the ADA in numerous capacities including Executive Director of the Greater Philadelphia Affiliate, National Director of Affiliate Development, Associate Executive Vice President for Operations, Deputy Executive Vice President and Chief Executive Officer. Before joining the American Diabetes Association, John served the Boy Scouts of America for nine years. John is a past Chair of the National Health Council's Board of Directors, and currently serves as a member of the Community Health Charities Board of Directors and the ASAE Foundation Board of Directors. He has a bachelor's degree from Franklin & Marshall College.

Jon Marie Hautz, CEBS is a Senior Consultant in the Health and Group Insurance Practice for William M. Mercer, Incorporated, an international human resources consulting company. There she assists companies in defining long-term healthcare benefit directions, assessing their current programs and implementing new health benefit strategies. Prior to Mercer, she was Director of Managed Care Plans for Federated Department Stores where she was responsible for the strategic direction and management of the employee healthcare benefit program covering over 45,000 active and retired employees. Her experience also includes designing and developing health insurance products for a large insurance company. She was the founding president of the Cincinnati/Dayton chapter of the International Society of Certified Employee Benefit Specialists (CEBS). She is vice president and board trustee for the Cincinnati Health Collaborative and was most recently vice president of the Employers Managed Health Care Association headquartered in Washington, DC. She holds a Bachelor of Science degree from the University of Louisville's School of Business.

George Isham, MD is medical director and chief health officer for HealthPartners. He is active in strategic planning and policy issues and coordinates and supports quality and medical management activities. He is a founding board member of and key liaison to the Institute for Clinical Systems Integration, a collaborative of Twin Cities medical groups that is implementing clinical practice guidelines. Dr. Isham provides leadership for *Partners for Better Health*, HealthPartners' program for improving the health of its members. Dr. Isham has been involved in quality measurement at the national and state levels. Currently, he co-chairs National Committee on Quality Assurance's (NCQA) committee on performance measurement which oversees the Health Employer Data and Information Set (HEDIS). Dr. Isham is a member of the board of directors of the Minnesota Health Data Institute, a public-private partnership to produce health care quality information for Minnesota. Dr. Isham is a past member of the board of directors of the American Association of Health Plans, a trade association of more than 1000 HMOs, PPOs and similar health plans. He serves on the U.S. Task Force on Community Preventive Services and the Institute of Medicines' Board of Health Promotion and Disease Prevention. Before his current position, Dr. Isham was medical director for MedCenters Health Plan in Minneapolis. In the late 1980s, he was executive director for University Health Care, Inc., an organization affiliated with the University of Wisconsin in Madison. Dr. Isham received his master of science in preventive medicine/administrative medicine at the University of Wisconsin Madison, and his doctor of medicine degree from the University of Illinois. He completed his internship and residency in internal medicine at the University of Wisconsin Hospital and Clinics in Madison. His practice experience as a primary care physician included 8 years at the Freeport Clinic in Freeport, Illinois, and 3 1/2 years as clinical assistant professor in Medicine at the University of Wisconsin.

Gregg O. Lehman, PhD is President and CEO of the National Business Coalition on Health, and leads a movement of 100 business coalitions nationwide seeking cost effective, better quality healthcare for employees and their families. He oversees the effort to advance community-based health care reform by strengthening a national presence for local coalitions of employers that comprise NBCH's membership. Prior to joining NBCH Dr. Lehman gained valuable experience as CEO of Buyers Healthcare Cooperative in Nashville, TN. Dr. Lehman also served as Vice President of National Business Development for Vivra Health Advantage, a chronic disease management company also in Nashville, TN. His not-for-profit experience includes serving as President of the NFIB Foundation in Washington, D.C. and President of Taylor University, Upland, IN. In his current position, Dr. Lehman is actively working with coalitions to promote the role of coalitions in relation to national health policy and legislation. In addition, he is actively developing NBCH into an enterprise that assists local coalitions through the development of national contracts for products and services as well as strategic partnerships to further value-based health care purchasing and health care quality measurement. He earned a Ph.D. in Higher Education Administration, with a minor in Finance and Economics, at Purdue University.

Robert S. McDonough, MD is a medical director in Aetna Inc.'s MedicalPolicy and Transplant Department, where he is responsible for developing Aetna's coverage policies, clinical practice guidelines, preventive services guidelines, and continuing medical education monographs. He is co-chairman of Aetna's National Pharmacy and Therapeutics Committee. He has special interests in preventive health services, technology assessment, and outcomes research. He is former senior analyst and project director with the Health Program of the Congressional Office of Technology Assessment. He is a graduate of Duke University School of Medicine and School of Law (J.D.), and has a Masters degree in policy analysis from Duke's Sanford Institute of Public Policy. He completed an internship in internal medicine at Stanford University School of Medicine, and is a Fellow of the American College of Legal Medicine.

Dennis Scanlon, PhD is Assistant Professor of Health Policy and Administration in Penn State's Department of Health Policy & Administration. Dr. Scanlon received his Ph.D. from the University of Michigan and holds a Masters degree in economics from the University of Pittsburgh. Dr. Scanlon has authored several articles on health plan quality, performance measurement and quality improvement, consumer choice of health insurance plans, and health plan accreditation. Dr. Scanlon recently authored a value-purchasing guide, commissioned by the Agency for Healthcare Research and Quality (AHRQ), to help employers become 'catalysts for quality improvement.' In addition, Dr. Scanlon recently completed a federally funded research project examining the state of quality improvement activities at managed care plans, and the degree to which plans are using performance measures to improve quality.

Dr. Scanlon is currently working on a five-year program project with researchers at the University of California at San Francisco and the University of Michigan, examining the impact of competition on the quality of care provided by managed care organizations. This project is also funded by AHRQ. He is also working with several employers and health plans to assess the degree of variation and cost-effectiveness of disease management programs. Dr. Scanlon teaches undergraduate and graduate courses at Penn State on Managed Care, Health Economics, and Quantitative Methods for Health Services Research.

John Stevens, MD is interim Strategic Business Manager for the American Cancer Society's $116,500,000 Research and Health Professional Training Program and has been Vice President for Extramural Grants since 1988. In the latter capacity, he is responsible for managing the Society's $91,000,000 Research and Health Professional Training Grants portfolio, and the peer review system by which the 1,500 grant applications received annually by the Society are ranked in order of merit for funding. John also is a member of the Senior Management Team, which provides National staff with the strategic vision to achieve the Society's major goal of changing the course of the disease and setting the stage for controlling cancer early in the new century.

John received his MD degree from the University of Buenos Aires, Argentina, and joined the Society in 1981. Prior to that, he held a faculty appointment in the Biochemistry Department at the Mount Sinai School of Medicine of the City University of New York where he conducted research on steroid hormones and leukemia with grant support from the National Cancer Institute, the Leukemia Society of America, as well as the American Cancer Society.

Bruce Taylor, Director—Employee Benefit Policy and Plans, is responsible for the strategy and management of Verizon's healthcare and other welfare benefit plans. Mr. Taylor actively contributes to national healthcare issues through his participation in employer and healthcare organizations. He provided staff support to the President's Advisory Commission on Consumer Protection and Quality in the Health Care Industry and worked directly with the Commission's Subcommittee drafting the Consumer Bill of Rights and Responsibilities. Mr. Taylor currently serves on the Board of Directors of the Washington Business Group on Health, the American Benefits Council, the Dallas-Ft. Worth Business Group on

Health, the New York Business Group on Health, and as a Trustee of the Employer's Managed Healthcare Association (MHCA). He was also a founding member of The Leapfrog Group—all working to promote high quality, accountable, and cost-effective employee benefit programs. He previously served on the Employee Benefits Committee of the United States Independent Telephone Association and both the Health Care Subcommittee and the Employee Benefits Committee of the National Association of Manufacturers. He has been a frequent speaker on employee benefit financing and health cost management issues, and continuously "borrows" ideas from other employers and healthcare providers. He is a graduate of the University of Connecticut, The American College, and the University of New Haven.

Reed Tuckson, MD, a graduate of Howard University and Georgetown University School of Medicine, is currently Senior Vice President of Consumer Health and Medical Care Advancement at UnitedHealth Group. He has served as Senior Vice President, Professional Standards, for the American Medical Association (AMA). He is former President of the Charles R. Drew University of Medicine and Science in Los Angeles from 1991 to 1997; has served as Senior Vice President for Programs of the March of Dimes Birth Defects Foundation from 1990 to 1991; and from 1986 to 1990, Dr. Tuckson was the Commissioner of Public Health for the District of Columbia. He currently is a member of Institute of Medicine of the National Academy of Sciences and serves as a member of the Secretary of Health and Human Services' Advisory Committee on Genetic Testing and has held a number of other federal appointments, including cabinet level advisory committees on health reform, infant mortality, children's health, violence, and radiation testing.

Dale Whitney is Corporate Health and Welfare Manager at UPS and has responsibility for the health care and ancillary benefit programs for over 700,000 UPS employees, retirees and their families. Following several assignments in Operations, Health and Safety and Employment, Dale served as Human Resources Manager in several western states. He has been in the UPS Corporate Health and Welfare function for over ten years and moved to Atlanta with the UPS Corporate Office in 1991. Dale is a member of several national and local professional organizations and currently on the board of the Employers Managed Health Care Association in Washington. D.C. and a member of the National Committee for Quality Assurance (NCQA) Purchaser Advisory Council. He is also a board member of the Georgia Healthcare Leadership Council, a group of employers, health plans and health care providers that was recently named one of the initial sites to roll out the Leapfrog Group patient safety initiatives.

Appendix II

Speaker's Company Profiles

Aetna

Aetna provides managed care benefits and dental, pharmacy, vision, and group insurance coverage. Aetna covers more than 18 million individuals under its health plans, plus more than 14 million dental plan members and some 11 million group members. Aetna has radically restructured its operations by selling the Financial Services division and its international businesses to Dutch insurer ING Group, making Aetna strictly a health and related benefits company. Its annual revenues are approximately 24.7 billion dollars.

Agency for Healthcare Research and Quality

The Agency for Healthcare Research and Quality (AHRQ) is designed to support research design to improve the quality of health care, reduce its cost, improve patient safety, address medical errors, and broaden access to essential services. AHRQ sponsors and conducts research that provides evidence-based information on health care outcomes; quality; and cost, use and access. The information helps health care decision makers—patients and clinicians, health system leaders, and policymakers—make more informed decisions and improve the quality of health care services. In fiscal year 2001, AHRQ received an appropriation of approximately 270 million dollars.

American Association of Health Plans

The American Association of Health Plans (AAHP) is the nation's principal association of health plans, representing more than 1,000 plans that provide coverage for approximately 150 million Americans nationwide. Member plans include health maintenance organizations (HMOs), preferred provider organizations (PPOs), other similar health plans and utilization review organizations (UROs). AAHP's mission is to advance health care quality and affordability through leadership in the health care community, advocacy and the provision of services to member health plans.

American Cancer Society

Dedicated to the elimination of cancer, the American Cancer Society is a not-for-profit organization, staffed by professionals and more than 2 million volunteers at some 3,400 local units across the country. ACS is the largest source of private cancer research funds in the U.S. In addition to research, the ACS supports detection, treatment, and education programs. The organization encourages prevention efforts with programs such as the Great American Smokeout. Patient services include moral support, transportation to and from treatment, and camps for children who have cancer. Programs account for about 71% of expenses; 29% goes to administration and fund-raising.

American Diabetes Association

The American Diabetes Association is the nation's leading nonprofit health organization providing diabetes research, information and advocacy. Founded in 1940, the American Diabetes Association conducts programs in all 50 states and the District of Columbia, reaching more than 800 communities. The mission of the organization is to prevent and cure diabetes, and to improve the lives of all people affected by diabetes. To fulfill this mission, the American Diabetes Association funds research, publishes scientific findings, provides information and other services to people with diabetes, their families, health care professionals and the public and advocates for scientific research and for the rights of people with diabetes.

HealthPartners

HealthPartners is a family of nonprofit Minnesota health care organizations focused on improving the health of its members, its patients and the community. HealthPartners is consumer-governed. HealthPartners and its related organizations provided health care services, insurance and HMO coverage to nearly 660,000 members. More than 9,200 employees staff the various HealthPartners organization. HealthPartners family includes Group Health, a staff-model health maintenance organization (HMO) founded in 1957, and the former MedCenters Health Plan, a network-model HMO founded in 1972. HealthPartners affiliated with Regions Hospital, Ramsey clinics and Regions Hospital Foundation in 1993.

Marriott

Marriott International is the #1 lodging company in the world with almost 2,400 owned or franchised properties in 64 countries. Its hotel brands include Courtyard, Marriott, Residence Inn, Spring Hill Suites, and Ritz-Carlton. Other operations include Marriott Vacation Club International (time-share resorts), Marriott Senior Living Services (senior living communities), and Marriott Distribution Services (distribution of food and related items). The company was formed in 1998 when Marriott International split its lodging operations from its food and facilities management services (now run by Sodexho Alliance). The Marriott family owns about 18% of the company, and its revenues for fiscal year 2000 were approximately 9.4 billion dollars.

Medical Technology Leadership Forum

The Medical Technology Leadership Forum (MTLF) is a not-for-profit membership organization headquartered in Washington, DC. Founded in 1996, MTLF consists of a broad cross-section of the physicians, research institutions and universities, manufacturers, and patient organizations. Its mission is to provide a unified, multi-sectional voice for sustaining and enhancing technological innovation and to improve health outcomes and the quality of life for all Americans. To meet this goal MTLF works to educate the public, providers, and policy makers about the role of medical technology and the need to sustain technological innovation.

United Healthgroup

Operating through five segments, the company offers a variety of health care plans and services. Its United Healthcare segment manages HMO, PPO, and POS (point-of-service) plans; its Ovations unit focuses on providing Medicare and Medicaid options to enrollees over 50 (including the members of AARP). Uniprise handles health plans for large companies, and Specialized Care Services offers just that — vision care, dental care, transplant services, and other niche coverage. Ingenix provides health information consulting and publishing as well as drug development and marketing services. United Health operates nationwide, and has annual revenues of approximately 23.5 billion dollars.

United Parcel Service

The United Parcel Services is the world's #1 package-delivery company. Its operates throughout the US and more than 200 countries and territories. UPS is the leading ground-delivery firm and is gaining on rival FedEx in air delivery; it delivers nearly 14 million packages per day. Through UPS Logistics and UPS Consulting, the company is expanding its role in managing supply chain operations and logistics for corporations, and it has built a freight-forwarding business through acquisitions. UPS has also launched e-Ventures to develop operations supporting e-commerce. UPS had an income of approximately 30 billion dollars for fiscal year 2000. Managers, employees, retirees, and the founding families own 90% of UPS.

Verizon

Verizon was formed in 2000 when Bell Atlantic bought GTE, and is the #1 local phone company in the U.S. and the #2 telecom services provider, behind AT&T. Verizon has 62 million local-access lines throughout the U.S. Verizon Wireless, the company's joint venture with Vodafone, is the #1 U.S. wireless provider, with about 28.7 million mobile phone customers nationwide. Outside the U.S., Verizon affiliates serve 36 million wireless customers and operate 13 million access lines; the company also plans to build a multinational data network. Verizon has 6.9 million U.S. long-distance customers, and its revenues for fiscal year 2000 were approximately 68 billion dollars.

Wellmark

Wellmark Blue Cross and Blue Shield offers a full range of health insurance and related products and services and employs 1,723 people. As part of the Blue Cross Blue Shield Association, Wellmark is part of a national network of 46 plans that insure nearly 78 million Americans. Wellmark has 1.35 million customers in Iowa and South Dakota.

Appendix III

Purchaser Payer Background Information

Vanessa Walker

In 1999, the United States spent $1.2 trillion on health care, up 5.6% from the previous year.[1] Growth in health care expenditures is estimated to increase 8.3% in 2000 and 2001. Total spending on health insurance premiums was $401 billion in 1999, up 6.5% from the previous year. Total spending for clinical research is estimated at over $13.4 billion for 2000.[2] This estimate includes private sector spending on phase I-IV clinical trials ($6.7 billion in 1999) and NIH reported clinical research spending. Of the $5.3 billion NIH spends on clinical research an estimated $1.9 billion is spent on clinical trials. Other government agencies add at most $1.4 billion dollars (including: Veterans Affairs, Department of Defense, Agency for Healthcare Research and Quality, Centers for Disease Control, Health Resources and Services Administration, and Centers for Medicare and Medicaid Services, and Food and Drug Administration).

A recent New York Times article noted that large insurance companies observed medical cost increases of 10 to 15 percent in Q1 2001 roughly more than double the 5-6 percent increase seen in the past decade.[3] Preliminary estimates from Hewitt Associates show that HMOs are requesting premium in-

---

[1] Heffler S, Levit K, Smith S, Smith C, Cowan C, Lazenby H, and Freeland M. Health Spending up in 1999; Faster Growth Expected in the Future. Health Affairs 20(2): 193–232. 2001

[2] PHRMA. Pharmaceutical Industry Profile 2001. Washington, DC: 2001

[3] Milt Freudenheim. "Medical Costs Surge as Hospitals Force Insurers to Raise Payments." New York Times, 5/25/01.

creases averaging 18.3 percent, with some proposed increases reaching as high as 60 percent.

In 1999, *Health Affairs* reported health insurance premiums increased 6.5% in 1999, faster than the period between 1993 and 1998, which averaged 5.0% annual growth. In that same year, health insurance premiums totaled $401.2 billion spent on health, while $355.3 billion was spent on benefits. The article predicted that premiums would continue to increase 9.3% in 2000, and 10.5% in 2001. During this period, it was believed that premium growth would surpass benefit growth.[4]

Also noted in the article, hospitals are requesting double-digit rate increase from insurers due to growing labor and utility costs in 2000 and 2001. Insurers are, in turn, passing additional costs from hospitals and other providers to employers in the form of increased premiums averaging 18%.

Spending on prescription drugs rose 16.2% in 2000.[5] The fastest-growing categories of drugs in terms of number of prescriptions written were antihistamines (18.4% increase), cholesterol-lowering drugs (18.1%) and antidepressants (11.3%). Factors influencing health care costs include:

- Aging population
- Diminished competition (mergers of providers and insurers)
- Increased medical inflation
- Increased prescription drug costs
- Strong demand for medical services
- Growth in technology including information technology investments

The top disease categories based on cost or utilization indicators include: Cancer, Ischemic heart disease, Congestive Heart Failure, Injury, Complications of Medical and Surgical care, Complications of Pregnancy, Psychiatric Conditions, and Asthma (Table 1).

A survey of 20 licensed HMO plans that published research in the public domain and had a specific infrastructure to support research, had 1996 revenue of $92 million and employed 1,273 staff.[6] The selected plans covered more than 29 million members. Research conducted by these entities included health services, epidemiology, health economics, and clinical trials. The plan or parent organization and NIH were the largest source of funds (24% and 22%, respectively).

---

[4] Heffler, et al.

[5] Express Scripts. Express Scripts 2000 drug trend report. St. Louis. MO: June, 2001

[6] Neslon AF, Quiter ES, Solberg LI. The state of Research within Managed Care Plans 1997 Survey. Health Affairs 17(1): 128–138.

TABLE 1 Ranking of Top 16 Principal Diagnosis Disease Cohorts*

Condition	Ranking of Total allowed dollars	Ranking of Total allowed dollars per patient per year	Ranking of Admits per patient per year	Ranking of ER visits per patient per year
Cancer	1	2	10	16
Ischemic Heart Disease	2	4	4	12
Other Heart Disease	3	5	5	11
Injury	4	13	15	1
Congestive Heart Failure	5	1	1	8
Diabetes	6	10	9	6
Congestive Obstructive Pulmonary Disease	7	9	7	7
Complications of Medical and Surgical Care	8	3	3	5
Arthropathies	9	14	13	14
Dorsopathies	10	12	14	9
Psychiatric conditions	11	11	12	4
Disease of Liver, Pancreas	12	8	8	10
Disorder of Female Genital Organs	13	16	16	15
Cerebrovascular Disease	14	6	6	13
Complication of Pregnancy	15	7	2	3
Asthma	16	15	11	2

*Data from a large Commercial and Medicare+Choice HMO population in 2000 in the southeastern United States. Members may appear in more than one category.

Appendix IV

Workshop Agenda

DECEMBER 12, 2001
Park Hyatt Hotel, Washington, DC
Park Hyatt Ballroom

8:30 am **Welcoming Remarks and Meeting Objectives**

Clinical Research Roundtable Co-Chairs

Enriqueta Bond, Ph.D.
President
Burroughs Welcome Fund

William Gerberding, Ph.D.
President Emeritus
University of Washington

Workshop Co-Chairs

Allan Korn, M.D.
Senior Vice President and Chief Medical Officer
Blue Cross Blue Shield Association

Sean Tunis, M.D., M.Sc.
Director, Coverage and Analysis Group
Office of Clinical Standards and Quality
Centers for Medicare and Medicaid Services

9:00 **Purchaser Perspective**

Each speaker has been asked to present a brief 5 min. overview of their responses to the two broad questions.

Moderator—Patricia Salber MD, General Motors

Jill Berger
Corporate Health and Welfare
  Manager
Marriot

Dale Whitney
Corporate Health and Welfare
  Manager
United Parcel Service

Helen Darling
President
Washington Business Group on
Health

Gregg Lehman
President & CEO
National Business Coalition on
Health

Bruce Taylor
Director National Health Care &
  Policy Plans
Verizon

Jon Hautz
Senior Consultant
William M. Mercer Inc.

9:30 Clinical Research Roundtable Discussion

10:15 Questions and Comments from the Audience

10:30 **Break**

10:45 **Payer & Health System Perspective**

Each speaker has been asked to present a brief 5 min. overview of their responses to the two broad questions.

Moderators—Alan Korn, Blue Cross Blue Shield Association and Sean Tunis, Centers for Medicare and Medicaid Services

Eric Book, MD
Chief Medical Officer
Wellmark

Reed Tuckson, MD
Chief Medical Officer
United Healthgroup

Robert McDonough, MD
Medical Director for Quality
  Management
Aetna

George Isham, MD
Medical Director and Chief Health
  Officer
HealthPartners

Chuck Cutler, MD
Chief Medical Officer
American Association of Health
  Plans

11:15	Clinical Research Roundtable Discussion
12:00	Questions and Comments from the Audience
12:15 pm	**Lunch (for members and guests in the meeting room)**
1:15	**Stakeholder Perspective**

Please respond to the issues raised in the first two panels. What are your needs? What is your role? What can you contribute to the Clinical Research Enterprise?

Moderator—Myrl Weinberg, President, National Health Council

Francis Chesley, MD
Director, Office of Research, Review, Education and Policy Agency for Healthcare, Research & Quality

Susan Foote, JD
Board Member, Medical Technology Leadership Forum

Dennis Scanlon, Ph.D.
Associate Professor, Health Policy and Administration Pennsylvania State University

Robert M. Califf, MD
Division of Cardiology, Department of Medicine Duke University

John H. Graham IV
Chief Executive Officer American Diabetes Association

John Stevens, MD
Vice President for Extramural Grants Research Department American Cancer Society

1:45	Clinical Research Roundtable Discussion
2:30	Questions and Comments from the Audience
2:45	**Break**
3:00	**Roundtable Discussion: Opportunities and challenges**

This two-hour discussion regarding opportunities and challenges for the Clinical Research Enterprise will begin with a 20-minute presentation by Dr. Lou Sherwood. Audience participation is welcome.

Moderators—Allan Korn, BCBSA and Sean Tunis, CMS

"The Second Frontier" – Lou Sherwood, M.D.
Senior Vice President for Medical and Scientific Affairs
Merck and Company

5:00   **Concluding Remarks**

Enriqueta Bond, Ph.D.
President
Burroughs-Welcome Fund

William Gerberding, Ph.D.
President Emeritus
University of Washington

Appendix V

Definitions of Clinical Research and Components of the Enterprise

DEFINITION OF CLINICAL RESEARCH

(Clinical Research: A National Call to Action, November 1999) Clinical research is a component of medical and health research intended to produce knowledge valuable for understanding human disease, preventing and treating illness, and promoting health. Clinical Research embraces a continuum of studies involving interactions with patients, diagnostic clinical materials or data, or populations in any of the following categories: (1) disease mechanisms (etiopathogenesis); (2) bi-directional integrative (translational) research; (3) clinical knowledge, detection, diagnosis and natural history of disease; (4) therapeutic interventions including development and clinical trials of drugs, biologics, devices, and instruments; (5) prevention (primary and secondary) and health promotion; (6) behavioral research; (7) health services research, including outcomes, and cost-effectiveness; (8) epidemiology; and (9) community-based and managed care-based trials.

MAJOR COMPONENTS OF THE CLINICAL RESEARCH ENTERPRISE

Sponsors

Sponsors include private and public sector funding organizations such as the National Institutes of Health, pharmaceutical companies, medical device manufacturers, biotechnology firms, universities, private foundations, and national societies. Within the public sector the National Institutes of Health (NIH) is the largest clinical research sponsor, followed by the Department of Defense (DOD), the Department of Veterans Affairs (VA), Agency for Healthcare Research and Quality (AHRQ), and the Centers for Disease Control (CDC).

Research Organizations

Research organizations include academic health centers, private research institutes, survey research organizations, federal government intramural research programs, and contract research organizations.

Investigators

Investigators are the scientists performing clinical research from varied disciplines with a range of academic qualifications (e.g., MD, Ph.D., RN, DDS, PharmD).

Participants

Participants are the human volunteers, medical information and biological materials of human origin, or data derived from volunteers. Participants may have particular health conditions or may be healthy volunteers or populations at large.

Oversight Entities

Oversight entities include Institutional Review Boards, Food and Drug Administration, Department of Health and Human Services, Veterans Affairs, National Committee for Quality Assurance, and other national regulatory agencies.

Stakeholders/Consumers

Stakeholders/Consumers include health insurers, managed care organizations, health care systems, organized medicine, voluntary health agencies, patient advocacy groups, purchasers of health care, and providers of health care, public health systems, and individual consumers.

Appendix VI

Registered Workshop Participants

Elizabeth Adams
Sr. Director of Clinical and Research Projects

Sousan Altaie
Food and Drug Administration

Rochelle Archuleta
David Winston Health Policy Fellowship

Ivy Baer
Association of American Medical Colleges

Eileen Barker
FDA

Melissa Bartlett
American Medical Group Assoc.

Donna Bergeson
Alston & Bird LLP

Erica Bisguier-Reed
The Health Strategies Consultancy LLC

Patricia Brandt
National Institutes of Health

June Bray
Forum for Collaboration HIV Research

Katherine Browne
Academy for Health Services Research and Health Policy

Suanna Bruinooge
American Society of Clinical Oncology

Marguerite Burns
University of Wisconsin Medical School

Sarah Callahan
Academy for Health Services Research and Health Policy

Michael Campbell

Edward Campion
New England Journal of Medicine

David Chambers
National Institute of Mental Health

Cheryl Chanaud
University of Texas Medical Branch

Michael Chanin
Powell, Goldstein, Frazer & Murphy LLP

Lanhee Chen
The ERISA Industry Committee

Azhar Choudhry
Clinical Data Associate

Joel Cohen
AHRQ

J.C. Comolli
Center on AIDS and Other Medical Consequences of Drug Abuse, National Institute on Drug Abuse, National Institutes of Health

Rosaly Correa-de-Araujo, MD, MSc, PhD
American Society of Consultant Pharmacists

Toni D'Agostino
University of Texas Medical Branch

Hassan Danesi
Doctor

Andrea Denicoff
National Cancer Institute

Sally Duran
Mid Atlantic Medical Services, Inc. (MAMSI)

Marc Ehman, MPH
Institute of Medicine

Lisa Evans
U.S. Department of Health and Human Services

JoAnna Farrell
Centers for Medicare and Medicaid Services

Ellen Feigal
Division of Cancer Treatment and Diagnosis, National Cancer Institute, National Institutes of Health

Pamela Ebert Flattau
Flattau Associates, LLC

Sara Froelich
American Medical Group Assoc.

John Gallin
NIH

Karen Gervais
Minnesota Center for Health Care Ethics

Robin Goracke
Legislative Assistant
Rep. C. Peterson

VI: REGISTERED WORKSHOP PARTICIPANS

Maureen Gormley
Warren Grant Magnuson Clinical Center

Warren Greenberg
Scholar-in-residence AHRQ
George Washington University

John Greene
National Association of Health Underwriters

Albert Guay
American Dental Association

Kim Gunter
PricewaterhouseCoopers

Penny Hodgson
Duke Clinical Research Group

Scott Hunt
The Endocrine Society

John Iglehart
Health Affairs

Edward Im
Trigon Blue Cross Blue Shield

Joseph Jackson
Bristol-Myers Squibb

Wendy Johnson-Taylor
NIH, Division of Nutrition Research Coordination

Aranthan Jones II
National Institutes of Health

Sharon Karnash
Duke Clinical Research Group

Sophia Kazakova
Johns Hopkins SPH

Sherry Keramidas
Regulatory Affairs Professionals Society

Catharine A. Kopac
Georgetown Medical Center, Center for Clinical Bioethics

Theodore Kotchen
Medical College of Wisconsin

Michael Lacey
Boston Scientific Corp

Wendy Landow
CIRREF

Denys Lau
Johns Hopkins / AHRQ

Dr. Matthew Liang
Brigham & Women's Hospital

Michael Mabry
SCVIR

Linda Magno
American Hospital Association

Scott Marchand
National Cancer Institute

John McDermott
Covance Health Economics and Outcomes Services, Inc.

Timothy McDonald
Fuqua School of Business, Duke University

Peggy McNamara
Agency for Healthcare Research and Quality

Dan Mendelson
Health Strategies LLC

John Miller
Maryland Health Care Coalition

Nancy E. Miller
Office of the Director, NIH

Barbara Myklebust
George Washington University

Dr. Ruth Nowjack-Raymer
National Institute of Dental and Craniofacial Research

Chuke Nwachuku
National Heart, Lung and Blood Institute

Karen Oliver
National Institute of Mental Health

Tina Ommaya
Covance Health Economics and Outcomes Services, Inc.

Ginger Penick Parra
National Health Policy Forum

Vaishali Patel
Johns Hopkins School of Public Health

Susana Perry
U.S. Administration on Aging

Paul Pomerantz
Society of Cardiovascular & Interventional Radiology

G. Gregory Raab
Consultant

Randel Richner
Boston Scientific Corp

R. Lucia Riddle
Principal Financial Group

Dallas Salisbury
Employee Benefit Research Inst.

Adam L. Scheffler, MA LSW
Health Policy Researcher

Clifford Schold
University of Pittsburgh

Michele Schoonmaker
FDA/CDRH/DLCD

Julie Scott
American Dental Association

Steven Sheingold
Centers for Medicare and Medicaid Services

Lawrence Shulman
National Institutes of Health

Yasmin Sivji
Doctor